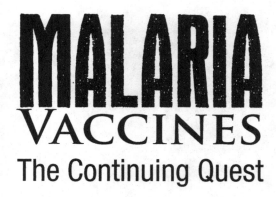

MALARIA
VACCINES
The Continuing Quest

MALARIA
VACCINES
The Continuing Quest

Irwin W Sherman
Division of Host-Microbe Systems & Therapeutics
School of Medicine
University of California at San Diego

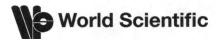

World Scientific

:W JERSEY · LONDON · SINGAPORE · BEIJING · SHANGHAI · HONG KONG · TAIPEI · CHENNAI · TOKYO

Published by

World Scientific Publishing Europe Ltd.
57 Shelton Street, Covent Garden, London WC2H 9HE
Head office: 5 Toh Tuck Link, Singapore 596224
USA office: 27 Warren Street, Suite 401-402, Hackensack, NJ 07601

Library of Congress Cataloging-in-Publication Data
Names: Sherman, Irwin W., author.
Title: Malaria vaccines : the continuing quest / Irwin W. Sherman.
Description: New Jersey : World Scientific, 2016
Identifiers: LCCN 2015048900 | ISBN 9781786340047 (hc : alk. paper)
Subjects: | MESH: Malaria--drug therapy | Malaria--parasitology | Malaria Vaccines |
    Adjuvants, Immunologic | Antigens, Protozoan
Classification: LCC RC157 | NLM WC 770 | DDC 616.9/36206--dc23
LC record available at http://lccn.loc.gov/2015048900

British Library Cataloguing-in-Publication Data
A catalogue record for this book is available from the British Library.

Desk Editors: Harini/Mary Simpson

Typeset by Stallion Press
Email: enquiries@stallionpress.com

Printed in Singapore

Contents

Preface   vii

Chapter 1.   The Three Lives of the Malaria Parasite   1

Chapter 2.   A Personal Scientific Odyssey   25

Chapter 3.   Taming the Malaria Parasite   63

Chapter 4.   The Quest for a Blood Stage Vaccine Begins   67

Chapter 5.   Malaria Vaccines and Malfeasance   77

Chapter 6.   Dreaming of a Nobel Prize   93

Chapter 7.   Molecular Biology Assists in Vaccine Development   99

Chapter 8.   Developing Vaccines against Blood Stages   115

Chapter 9.   PfEMP1, pfalhesin, and DBR   151

Chapter 10. Vaccines to Halt Transmission   173

Chapter 11. Sporozoite Invasion and the Path to RTS, S   189

Chapter 12.   Attenuated Plasmodial Vaccines   215

Chapter 13.   Viruses and Plasmodial Vaccines   225

Chapter 14.   Why the Quest Continues   231

References   237
Index   259

Preface

Malaria is the most important parasitic disease of humankind. About 3.4 billion — half the world's population — are at risk of malaria. It is transmitted in 108 countries, afflicts 216 million people, and each year causes 655,000 deaths.[1] Roughly 2,000 people die each day, mostly children under the age of five. Although most of the people of Asia and the Americas now live in areas where the risk of malaria is low, serious problems remain in economically underdeveloped areas and countries affected by social disruption. Of great concern is that there are malaria infections occurring in places once free of the disease. Over the years, the malaria parasite, *Plasmodium*, has become resistant to a variety of medicines, and often the best are either not available or too expensive for millions of people in developing nations. Further exacerbating the problem is insecticide resistance by the mosquitoes that transmit the parasite as well as economic constraints. Some believe a malaria vaccine is our only hope to eradicate the disease.

Although the first attempt at a malaria vaccine was made a century ago, it is only in the recent past that various malaria vaccine candidates have been tested in the hope of discovering a molecule that can provide long-lasting protection against the disease. Indeed, in late July of 2014, GlaxoSmithKline (GSK) announced that after 30 years of effort and an investment of $350 million, it has applied for regulatory approval for the world's first vaccine against malaria designed for children in Africa. In the development of this vaccine, called RTS, S, the Bill and Melinda Gates

Foundation provided more than $200 million in grant monies through its PATH Malaria Vaccine Initiative (MVI) for financial, scientific, managerial and field expertise. Because the effectiveness of RTS, S is ~30% it is clearly not the final answer to eradicating malaria. This book chronicles the development of RTS, S as well as the other investigations to find a more effective malaria vaccine. The quest for malaria vaccines has been enlivened by controversy; there have been wars of words, clashes of egos, and even a scandal or two. Errors have been made, ideas have been stolen, and credit for discovery has, at times, been unacknowledged. It has been a privilege to count myself as one among many investigators who have sought to find a malaria vaccine.

My hope is that this revised and updated version of The Elusive Malaria Vaccine: Miracle or Mirage? (ASM Press, 2009) will serve as a convenient and easily accessible source of information for students, teachers, microbiologists, parasitologists, physicians, clinicians, funders of research, as well as those who may want to redirect their research into malaria vaccines. And, finally in the telling of this continuing quest — the good and the bad, the ugly and the beautiful, the successes and the failures — I have tried to give the reader some insight into the creative process of scientific research.

Irwin W. Sherman

University of California at San Diego

Chapter 1

The Three Lives of the Malaria Parasite

Historically, the most common experience with malaria was that it was a sickness associated with wetlands. Indeed, the French name *paludisme* is from the Latin *"palus"* meaning swamp.[2] The name of the disease, literally 'bad air' comes from the belief that it resulted from human exposure to the poisonous vapors (miasma) that had seeped in from the polluted soil. But by the middle of the 19th century — a time when Louis Pasteur's germ theory was in full flower — there were various reports of a sighting of the causative agent of malaria. In 1879 two investigators in Italy, Edwin Klebs and Corrado Tommasi-Crudeli, found a bacillus in the mud and waters of the marshes in the highly malarious region of the Roman Campagna.[2] These bacteria when injected into rabbits resulted in fever, and the spleen was enlarged. They named the bacillus *Bacillus malariae*.

In the United States, the U.S. Board of Health commissioned Major George Sternberg, a well-trained bacteriologist, to try to repeat the experiments of Klebs and Tommasi-Crudeli in the malaria affected area around New Orleans.[2] He found bacteria similar to *B. malariae* in the mud from the Mississippi delta; however, after the bacteria were injected into rabbits the fevers produced were not typical of malaria in that they were not periodic. Sternberg was also able to produce the disease in rabbits by injecting them with his own saliva. He concluded that the disease was septicemia, not malaria, and suggested the bacteria were contaminants. What then was the cause?

1

i. Laveran's Animalcule

One of the signal characteristics of malaria in cadavers is the enlarged and blackened spleen and liver. This discoloration is the result of the accumulation of a brownish-black pigment. In 1847 the German pathologist–psychiatrist Heinrich Meckel, after observing the accumulation of pigment in the blood of a malaria patient with an enlarged spleen, proposed that the pigment itself, called hemozoin, was the cause of the disease.[3] L. F. Achille Kelsch (1841–1911), a pathologist working in malaria-ridden Algeria had been drawn to the pigment, and like Meckel he observed that hemozoin was almost always contained in the white blood cells but occasionally was enclosed in a clear body. In the main, Kelsch studied malaria in autopsied material but on occasion was able to examine blood from patients living with malaria and in almost all cases there was the telltale pigment. Although he recognized the presence of pigment as diagnostic for malaria and even found that the pigment appeared in the blood at the time of fever, Kelsch did not discover the causal agent itself.[2] Why? As a pathologist Kelsch looked at only dead material, and even freshly drawn blood would routinely be 'fixed' before microscopic examination: hence his failure.

Charles-Louis Alphonse Laveran (1845–1922) studied at the Public Health School in Strasbourg where he received his medical degree (1867). In 1874 after a competitive examination he was appointed Chair of Military Diseases and Epidemics at the Ecole du Val-de-Grace in Paris.[4] At Val-de-Grace Laveran became well acquainted with several physicians who had previously worked in the French territory of Algeria studying malaria. One in particular, L. F. Achille Kelsch exercised a profound influence on the young Laveran teaching him about the characteristics of malaria. Laveran has been described as "bespectacled with sharp features and a small trim beard." He was reputed to be extraordinarily precise, meticulous, singularly sharp-minded, incisive, and self-opinionated.[5] In short, he did not suffer fools gladly. Initially, in Algeria, Laveran spent much of his time looking at autopsy material (as did Kelsch) but he also examined fresh specimens. His microscope was not a good one and he used no stains but he was patient and determined. On November 6, 1880 while examining a drop of fresh blood, liquid and unstained from a feverish artilleryman he saw several transparent mobile filaments — flagella — emerging from a clear spherical body. He recognized that these bodies were alive, and that he was looking at an animal, not a bacterium or a fungus. Subsequently he examined blood samples from 192 malaria patients: in 148 of these he found telltale hemozoin-containing crescents.[6] Where there were no crescents, there were no symptoms of malaria. Laveran also found spherical bodies in or on the blood cells of those suffering with malaria all containing malaria pigment. He named the parasite *Oscillaria malariae* and communicated his findings to the Société Médicale des Hôspitaux on December 24, 1880. The drawings in his paper provide convincing evidence that, without use of stains or a microscope fitted with an oil immersion lens, Laveran had seen the development of the malaria "animalcule."

Laveran was anxious to confirm his observations on malaria parasites in other parts of the world, and so he traveled to the Santo Spirito Hospital in Rome where he met with two Italian malariologists (one of whom was Ettore Marchiafava, Tommasi-Crudeli's assistant and the other Angelo Celli, Professor of Hygiene) and showed them his slides. The Italians, whose chief interest was *B. malariae*, were unconvinced and told him that the spherical bodies he had seen were nothing more than degenerating red blood cells caused by *B. malariae* or some other cause.[2]

The vast majority of the medical world remained skeptical of Laveran's findings. In 1883 Marchiafava and Celli claimed to have seen the same bodies as described by Laveran but without any pigment granules. They also denied the visit by Laveran two years earlier. The Italians were unsuccessful in growing the bodies outside the body of the malaria patient. This lack of consensus on the causative agent was due not only to differences in interpretation of what was seen with the microscope, it was a matter of focus: the Italians emphasized the smallest forms in the blood, whereas Laveran concentrated on the hemozoin-laden crescents and the whip-like filaments.[2] While the search for the parasite itself occupied most research during this period, there was a serendipitous finding of great significance: malaria was an infectious disease, but not one that could be contracted by simply being exposed to a patient with a fever, as would be the case in persons with influenza. In 1882, C. Gerhardt deliberately induced malaria for therapeutic purposes in two patients with tertiary syphilis by injection of blood from another patient suffering with intermittent fever, and then cured them all with quinine. A year later Marchiafava and Celli, working on the wards of Rome's Santo Spirito Hospital, gave multiple injections intravenously and subcutaneously to five healthy subjects. Parasites were recovered from three of the five who came down with malaria; all recovered after quinine treatment. Clearly, it was the blood of a malaria patient that was infectious, not his breath.

In late 1884 or early 1885, Marchaifava and Celli abandoned their use of fixed stained smears and began to study, as had Laveran, fresh blood. Examining drops of liquid blood they observed the ameba-like movements of the parasite within the red blood cell and hence they called it *Plasmodium* (from the Latin *'plasmo'* meaning 'mold'). They also witnessed emerging whip-like filaments (called flagella) from the clear spherical bodies within the red blood cell although they questioned the significance of the flagella in the disease. The differences between the interpretations of Laveran and Marchiafava and Celli are now evident: for several years the Italians examined only dried stained specimens and so did not see any movement of the parasite that had caused Laveran to give it the name *Oscillaria*.[2]

Later, using both fixed, stained, and liquid preparations Marchaifava and Celli were able to trace the development of the small non-pigmented bodies within the red cell; they also described the hemozoin as the by-product of the destruction of the red cell's hemoglobin by the growing parasite. In 1886 during a visit to Europe Major George Sternberg visited Celli at the Santo Spirito Hospital. Celli drew a drop of blood from the finger of a malaria patient and was able to show Sternberg the ameba-like movement of the parasite and the emergence of flagella.[2] Sternberg returned to the United States and working with blood taken from a malaria patient in the Bay View Hospital in Baltimore was able to find Laveran's parasite in Welch's laboratory at Johns Hopkins University. A year later Welch separated the two kinds of malarias with 48 hour fever peaks; one would be named *P. vivax* and the other he named *Plasmodium falciparum* because it had sickle shaped crescents (and *'falcip'* in Latin means 'sickle or scythe').

In 1885, Camillo Golgi (1843–1926) of the University of Pavia convinced by the Italian confirmation of Laveran's observations felt malaria parasites deserved further study.[6] Examining the blood of 22 patients with a 72 hour fever cycle (later named *P. malariae*) he traced the tiny, unpigmented bodies of Marchiafava over three days until they grew to fill the red cell, and on the day of the fever paroxysm he found the pigment to concentrate in the center of the parasite as it divided. Golgi discovered that the parasite reproduced asexually by fission and correlated the clinical course of fever with destruction of the red blood cell to release the parasite. In 1886 when he noted that in both the 48 hour and the 72 hour fevers there were no crescents he effectively had distinguished the three kinds (species) of malaria based on fever symptoms. Marchiafava and his student, Amico Bignami, took Golgi's studies of malaria a step further. Although cases of 48 hour and 72 hour fever cycle malarias occurred throughout the year in Italy, in the autumn and summer they were outnumbered by a much more severe 48 hour-type, called aestivo-autumnal or malignant malaria. Only later, would it be recognized that the malignant disease was caused by the malaria parasite with crescents, *P. falciparum.*

Clinicians in the United States, however, continued to be skeptical of the significance of Laveran's discovery to malaria as a disease. William Osler, the premier blood specialist of his day, on hearing a paper presented at the inaugural meeting of the American Association of Physicians (June 1886) by W. T. Councilman, working in Welch's Johns Hopkins University laboratory, in which he found flagellated parasites in 80 attempts, challenged his findings. Osler also questioned the role of the flagellated bodies of Laveran, finding them improbable and contrary to all past experience of flagellated organisms occurring in the blood. By late 1886, however, after verifying the existence of the parasites with his own eyes — and postponing his Canadian vacation to examine the blood of every malaria patient he could find — Osler became a convert to the doctrine of "Laveranity." Osler published his findings on October 28, 1886 and in his 1889 treatise *Hematozoa of Malaria.* Henry Van Dyke Carter, a pathologist working at the Grant Medical College in India read Osler's paper. Previously, VanDyke Carter had been unable to find the malaria parasite in the blood, but with Osler's guidance he succeeded. Van Dyke Carter published his findings of three kinds of malaria parasites in India but for more than a decade his report received little notice among his colleagues in the Indian Medical Service. Despite this, malaria parasites were now being identified elsewhere: in Russia by Metchnikoff, by Morado and Coronado in Cuba, Anderson in Mauritius, and Atkinson in Hong Kong. By 1890 almost all the world believed in both the existence of Laveran's "animalcules" as well as in their being the cause of the disease malaria. The significance of Laveran's observation of the release of motile filaments (flagella) called exflagellation — would remain unappreciated, however, until William MacCallum and Eugene Opie of Johns Hopkins University made some critical observations.[2]

MacCallum and Opie were both medical students at Johns Hopkins when they followed up Laveran's observations using the malaria-like parasites found in the blood of birds. In 1897, Opie described some of these parasites in wild caught birds. During that same summer MacCallum, on vacation outside of Toronto, Canada studied one of these "malarias" named *Haemoproteus* where the male and female sex cells (gametocytes) in the blood are clearly different from one another even in unstained preparations. This is unlike human malarias where the gametocytes are very similar in appearance. One type, the hyaline or clear form put out Laveran's flagella, whereas the granular forms freed themselves from the red cell and remained quiescent. Observing the two forms in the same field under the microscope, he found the released flagella to invade and unite with the hyaline form to produce a wormlike gliding form. MacCallum immediately recognized that the flagella were sperm-like, that the granular forms were egg-like, and that he had witnessed fertilization to form a vermicule (later called the ookinete). On his return to Baltimore MacCallum confirmed his discovery in a woman suffering from subtertian (falciparum) malaria. In his 1898 publication MacCallum described the ookinete: "the movement is slow and even ... with the pointed end forward. It can move in any direction readily ... Often it is seen to rotate continually along its long axis. The forward progression ... occurs with considerable force ... pushing directly through the obstacle. The ultimate fate and true significance of these forms is difficult to determine." But, then he incorrectly concluded: "it is reasonable to suppose ... it is the much sought resistant stage."[7]

ii. Miasma to Mosquito

Although Ronald Ross, a Surgeon-Major in the Indian Medical Service, was a most unlikely person to solve the puzzle of how humans "catch" malaria, he did so.[5] Ross was born on Friday, May 13, 1857, in the foothills of the Himalayas where his father was an officer in the British Army stationed in India, which, at that time, was a part of the British Empire. As a boy of eight, his parents shipped him to England to receive a proper British education. He was a dreamer and, although he liked mathematics, he preferred wandering around the countryside, observing and collecting plants, and animals. At Springhill Boarding School, which he attended from the age of 12, he began to write poetry, painted watercolors and thought of becoming an artist. But, his father insisted him to study medicine in preparation for entry into the Indian Medical Service. Therefore, at age 17, young Ronald began his medical studies. He was not a good student, not because of laziness, but because he had so many other interests and could not concentrate on medicine. He preferred composing music to learning anatomy, and wrote epic dramas rather than writing prescriptions. Publishers rejected these "great works," and so he had them printed at his own expense. He eventually did pass his medical examination (after failing the first time), worked as a ship's doctor and then entered the Indian Medical Service. Although India was rife with disease — there was malaria, plague, and cholera — Ross busied himself writing mathematical equations, took long walks, wrote poetry, played the violin, and studied languages. Occasionally he used his microscope to look at the blood of soldiers ill with malaria, but he found nothing. He shouted to all who could hear: "Laveran is wrong. There is no germ of malaria."[8]

In 1894 Ross returned to England on leave. By that time, he had spent 13 years in India and had few scientific accomplishments: he wrote a few papers on malaria for the Indian Medical Gazette and claimed (without any real evidence) that malaria was primarily an intestinal infection. His hunt for the way malaria was transmitted from person-to-person began on April 9, when the 37-year old Ross visited with the 50-year old Patrick Manson at his home at 21 Queen Street in London.

Manson (1844–1922) received his medical training at the University of Aberdeen (1866) and then served as Medical Officer (1871–1873) to the British-run Chinese Imperial Maritime Customs Office in Amoy, a subtropical port in China.[5] There he studied the transmission via mosquito of the worm that causes elephantiasis. Returning to England (1889) he developed a lucrative consulting practice and was also appointed Medical Advisor to the Colonial Office in London. At the time of Ross' visit Manson was physician to the Seaman's Hospital Society at Greenwich and a lecturer on Tropical Diseases at St. George's Hospital and Charing

Cross Hospital Medical Schools where he had access to malaria contracted by sailors and others in the tropical regions of West Africa and India. Manson was a dedicated and experienced clinician as well as an expert microscopist and he had been shown Laveran's "animalcule" by H.G. Plimmer (1856–1918) of the University of London who in turn had been able to see the parasite under the guidance of Marchiafava during a visit to Rome. In his primitive laboratory on the top story of his house, night after night Manson watched the release of Laveran's flagella from the crescent forms. At the Seaman's Hospital, Manson took a drop of fresh blood from a sailor ill with malaria and showed Ross Laveran's parasite peppered with the black–brown malaria pigment as well as the release of flagella. One day, as the two were walking along Oxford Street, Manson said: do you know Ross, I have formed the theory that mosquitoes carry malaria … the mosquitoes suck the blood of people sick with malaria … the blood has those crescents in it … they get into the mosquito stomach, shoot out those whips … the whips shake themselves free and get into the mosquito's carcass … where they turn into a tough form like the spore of an anthrax bacillus … the mosquitoes die … they fall into water … people drink a soup of dead mosquitoes and they become infected.[5]

Manson based this idea on his own clinical studies with elephantiasis. Working in China, Manson had shown that the microscopic blood stages of the worm i.e. the microfilaria when taken up by the mosquito (called the gnat of Amoy) continued to mature within the mosquito body. Then, believing in the current notion that mosquitoes feed only once in their lifetime, he postulated that the filaria escape into the water in which the mosquito dies; the worms were subsequently swallowed and in this way the human contracted the disease. Manson's idea was based on several false assumptions and analogies. One was the earlier report (1870) of Alexei Fedchenko working in central Asia, who had shown that the guinea worm, *Dracunculus*, when released into water, entered into a tiny one-eyed crustacean, *Cyclops*, which when swallowed in the drinking water resulted in infection. Moreover, Manson did not realize that mosquitoes could feed more than once in a lifetime and did not die in the water after their eggs were laid after a single feeding. Thus, a string of seemingly "logical" deductions led to Manson's presumption that malaria parasites must be transmitted by ingestion. Manson had concocted a romantic story that was mostly a guess on his part, but the younger and inexperienced Ross took it as fact.

Ross left England in March 1895, and reached Bombay a month later. In June 1895, encouraged by Manson's passionate plea, he captured various kinds of mosquitoes, although he had no clue what kind they were. He set up an experiment using the water in which an infected mosquito had laid her eggs, her young had been observed swimming, and in which the off-spring had been allowed to die. The water with its dead and decaying mosquitoes was then given to a volunteer to drink. The man came down with a fever but after a few days, no crescents could be found in his blood. The same experiment was repeated with two other men who were paid for their services. Failure again. It thus appeared that drinking water with mosquito-infected material did not produce the disease. Ross began to think that, perhaps, the mosquitoes had the disease, but that they probably gave it to human beings by biting them and not by being eaten. He began to work with patients whose blood contained crescent-shaped malaria parasites, and with mosquitoes bred from larvae. The first task was to get the mosquitoes to bite the patients. It was like looking for a needle in a haystack. There are more than 2,500 different kinds of mosquitoes and, at the time, there were no good means for identifying most of them. Initially, Ross worked mostly with the gray and striped-wing kind. Although when these mosquitoes were dissected, there were the whip-like flagella in the mosquito stomach no further development occurred. This result was no more informative than what Laveran had seen in a drop of blood on a microscope slide nearly 20 years earlier. Today, we understand (as Ross did not) why this was so: the gray mosquitoes are *Culex* and those with striped wings are *Aedes,* and these do not carry human malaria. No, the one that he should have used was the brown, spotted winged mosquito, *Anopheles*, but Ross did not recognize this for the entire year he dissected mosquitoes. Each mosquito dissection had required hours of effort at the microscope and yet his prodigious labors had yielded nothing more than thousands of mosquito carcasses.

Then, at the age of 40 and having spent 17 years in the Indian Medical Service, Ross turned from the insusceptible kind of mosquito to the susceptible, brown, spotted winged one. On August 16, 1897, his assistant brought him a bottle in which mosquitoes were being hatched from larvae. It contained "about a dozen big brown fellows, with fine tapered bodies hungrily trying to escape through the gauze covering of the flask which the angel of fate had given my humble retainer!"[9] He wrote: "my mind was blank with the August heat; the screws of the microscope were rusted with sweat from my forehead and hands, while the last remaining eyepiece was cracked. I fed them on Husein Khan, a patient who had crescents in his blood. There had been some casualties among the mosquitoes, and only three were left on the morning of August 20, 1897. One of these had died and swelled up with decay."[9] At 7 a.m., Ross went to the hospital, examined patients, attended to correspondence and dissected the dead mosquito, without result. Then — a significant reminder of one of those unknown quantities in the equation to be solved — he examined another. No result again. He wrote in his notebook: "at about 1 p.m., I determined to sacrifice the last mosquito. Was it worth bothering about the last one, I asked myself? And, I answered myself, better finish off the batch. A job worth doing at all is worth doing well. The dissection was excellent and I went carefully through the tissues, now so familiar to me, searching every micron with the same passion and care as one would have in searching some vast ruined palace for a little hidden treasure. Nothing. No, these new mosquitoes also were going to be a failure: there was something wrong with the theory. But the stomach tissues still remained to be examined — lying there, empty and flaccid, before me on the glass slide, a great white expanse of cells like a large courtyard of flagstones, each one of which must be scrutinized — half an hour's labor at least. I was tired and what was the use? I must have examined the stomachs of a 1,000 mosquitoes by this time. But the angel of fate fortunately laid his hand on my head, and I had scarcely commenced the search again when I saw a clear and almost perfectly circular outline before me of about 12 microns in diameter. The outline was too sharp, the cell too small to be an ordinary stomach cell of a mosquito. I looked a little further. Here was another, and another exactly similar cell. The afternoon was very hot and overcast; and I remember opening the diaphragm of the substage condenser of the microscope to admit more light and then changing the focus. In each of these, there was a cluster of small granules, black as jet, and exactly like the black pigment granules of the … crescents. I made little pen-and-ink drawings of the cells with black dots of malaria pigment in them. The next day, I wrote the following verses and sent these to my dear wife:

> Seeking his secret deeds
> With tears and toiling breath,
> I find thy cunning seeds,
> O million-murdering death."[9]

Here was the critical clue to the manner of transmission. Ross had shown that, four or five days after feeding on infected blood, the mosquito had wart like oocysts on its stomach. He did not know if these kept on growing, however, nor how the mosquitoes became infective. He planned to answer these questions shortly but, before that work could begin, Ross reported his findings to the *British Medical Journal* in a paper entitled "On some peculiar pigmented cells found in two mosquitoes fed on malarial blood." It appeared December 18, 1897.

Ross knew he could wrap up the unfinished work in a matter of a few weeks, but then was struck by a blow from the Indian Medical Service by being ordered to proceed to Calcutta — immediately. As soon as he arrived in Calcutta, he set his hospital assistants the task of hunting for the larvae and pupae of the brown, spotted winged mosquitoes. Soon he had a stock of these, and set about getting them to bite patients who were suffering from malaria. By flooding the ground outside the laboratory, he hoped to imitate rain puddles and with this he began to learn about mosquito breeding. "If I am not on the pigmented cells again in a week or two," he wrote to Manson, "my language will be dreadful."[10]

In Calcutta, Ross was given a small laboratory. There were two Indian assistants who had already been working there when he arrived, but they were old men and not very intelligent, so he engaged two younger men, Purboona and Mahomed Bux. Both of these he paid out of his own monies. Since there were not a large number of malaria cases in the Calcutta hospitals, Ross turned to something that Manson had suggested earlier: the study of mosquitoes and malaria, as seen in birds. Pigeons, crows, larks, and sparrows were caught and placed in cages on two old hospital beds. Mosquito nets were put over the beds and then, at night, infected mosquitoes were put under the nets. Before much time had passed the crows and pigeons were found to harbor malaria parasites in their blood; also, he found the pigmented cells, which he previously had spotted in the stomachs of mosquitoes that had been fed on infected larks. Ross became certain of the whole life history in the mosquito, except he had not actually seen the ookinetes, described by MacCallum, turning into oocysts. This was the last stage in the study. He found that the oocysts depended, as regards their size, exactly on the length of time since the mosquitoes had been fed on infected blood. They grew to their maximum size about six days after the mosquito had fed on infected blood. They left the stomach after this time, but he did not know what happened to them then.

One day, while studying some sparrows he found that one was quite healthy, another contained a few of the malaria parasites, and the third had a large number of parasites in its blood. Each bird was put under a separate mosquito net and exposed to a group of mosquitoes from a batch that had been hatched out from grubs in the same bottle. Fifteen mosquitoes were fed on the healthy sparrow; in their stomachs, not one parasite was found. Nineteen mosquitoes were fed on the second sparrow; every one of these contained some parasites, though, in some cases, not very many. Twenty insects were fed on the third, badly infected, sparrow; every one of these contained some parasites in their stomachs and some contained huge numbers.

Ross wrote in his *Memoirs*[9]: "this delighted me! I asked the medical service for assistance and a leave, but was denied this. I wanted to provide the final story of the malaria parasite for this meeting; but, I knew that time was very short. I still did not have the full details of ... the change from the oocysts in the mosquito's stomach into the stages that could infect human beings and birds. Then, I found that some of the oocysts seemed to have stripes or ridges in them; this happened on the 7th or 8th day after the mosquito had been fed on infected blood." He continued "I spent hours every day peering into the microscope. The constant strain on mind and eye at this temperature is making me thoroughly ill." He had no doubt these oocysts with the stripes or rods burst — but did not know what happened to them. He asked himself: if they burst, did they produce the same stages that infected human blood?

Then, on July 4, 1898, Ross got something of value. Near a mosquito's head, he found a large branch-looking gland. It led into the head of the mosquito. Ross mused, "it is a thousand to one that it is a salivary gland. Did this gland infect healthy creatures? Did it mean that if an infected mosquito fed off the blood of an uninfected human being or bird, then this gland would pour some of the parasites ... into the blood of the healthy creature?"

On July 21 and 22 of that year, Ross took some uninfected sparrows, allowed mosquitoes (which had been fed on malaria-infected sparrows) to bite them and then, within a few days, was able to show that the healthy sparrows had become infected. This was the proof — this showed that malaria was not conveyed by bad air. On July 25, now sure, he sent off a triumphant telegram to Patrick Manson, reporting the complete solution; three days later, Manson spoke at the British Medical Association meeting in Edinburgh, describing the long and painstaking research Ross had been carrying out for years past. Ross' findings were communicated on July 28, 1898, and published in the August 20th issue of *The Lancet* and the September 24th issue of the *British Medical Journal*.

iii. A Matter of Priority: Ross vs. Grassi

During the summer of 1896 Manson learned that Amico Bignami at the Santo Spirito Hospital in Rome had attacked his mosquito theory with one of his own, namely that the mosquito passed on the parasite in feeding, not dying. In this Bignami placed special emphasis on his inoculation experiments: transfusion of blood from a patient with periodic fever into healthy persons resulted in a disease that could be cured by quinine. Although Bignami did not isolate the parasite it was clear to him that the disease with which he was working was malaria. He reasoned that the mosquito acted in a fashion similar to a hypodermic needle giving the parasite direct entry into the blood. On hearing Bignami's claim Ross became angry and began to suspect that the Italians were beginning to steal Manson's ideas. That same year, after Ross had carried out studies that convinced him that Manson's hypothesis of infection by mosquito ingestion was incorrect, he wrote: "the belief is growing on me that the disease is communicated by the bite of the mosquito. What do you think?" Manson encouraged caution: "the parasite might not develop in any old mosquito. Possibly different species of mosquito may modify the malaria germ." Indeed, Manson was correct.

Ross had done most of his work with mosquitoes (the gray *Culex* and the brindled *Aedes*) that do not transmit human malaria. By October 1896, Ross agreed with Manson that the mosquitoes with which he was working were not the right kind. In the summer of 1897 after he began to use the brown, dapple-winged mosquito, he found that after their feeding on a patient with crescents in the blood these changed into pigment-bearing globules in the mosquito stomach and that over time these grew in size. The brown–black pigment in the globules was indistinguishable in color and shape from that found in finger blood from a malaria patient. Ross thought he was "on it" and believed (but did not prove) the pigmented cells had transformed from Laveran's flagellum. This occurred on August 20, 1897, a day Ross called "Mosquito Day." In September Ross wrote a short note on his observations and sent them to Manson for communication to the *British Medical Journal* under the title "On some peculiar pigmented cells found in two mosquitoes fed on malarial blood." Ross wrote Manson: "I really believe the problem is solved, though I don't like to say so … I have hardly restrained myself from writing "pigment" to you …" Manson replied to the letter on October 29, 1898: "and you have to thank the plasmodium that it is fool enough to carry its pigment along with it into the mosquito's tissues. Otherwise, I suppose you would not have spotted him."[10]

His transfer to Calcutta where there were very few clinical cases interrupted Ross' work on human malaria. At Manson's suggestion Ross began to work on the bird malaria *P. relictum* transmitted by *Culex* mosquitoes. These findings were communicated to Manson and the scientific world in July of 1898 when Manson spoke at the meeting of the British Medical Association meeting in Edinburgh and appeared in published form in the August and September issues of the *Lancet* and the *British Medical Journal* respectively. Later, that Summer Ross recognized that "one single experiment with crescents will enable me to bring human malaria into line with (bird malaria) — they are sure to be the same." But, he never did the experiment. He left India for good on February 16, 1899.

During the period 1894 and 1898 — a time when Ross was working alone in India — the Italians published virtually nothing except for the 1896 paper by Bignami. But by the middle of July of 1898 — a time when Ross' proof was complete and partly published — the Italians, led by Giovanni Battista Grassi, began to work in earnest on the transmission of malaria. Grassi received a medical degree from the University of Padua (1875) however he never practiced medicine and by the time the work on transmission began he held the Chair in Comparative Anatomy in Rome. He was world-renowned for his studies in zoology including unraveling the complex and mysterious life history of the eel (1887) as well as the roundworm *Strongyloides*; he was able to diagnose hookworm disease by finding eggs in the feces, identified fleas as vectors of dog and mouse tapeworms and wrote a monograph on the marine chaetognaths. As early as 1890, he had worked with bird malaria, and this led quite naturally to studies of human malaria; together with Amico Bignami and Antonio Dionisi at the Santo Spirito Hospital they attempted (in 1894) to determine whether mosquitoes from the malarious areas were transmitters of the disease. In this, they were unsuccessful.[2]

Grassi was small in stature and delicate but with a serious and forceful will. He had long, black, curly hair, beetling eyebrows, and an unkempt shaggy beard. He usually wore a battered felt hat, tattered clothes and dark, smoked glasses. He seemed to enjoy a good quarrel and was pleased when such an opportunity presented itself. He was also very proud of the research he did and was resentful of those who questioned his authority.[5] Grassi recognized that insofar as malaria was concerned there remained two main tasks: demonstrate the developmental cycle of the human parasite in the mosquito and identify the kind of mosquito that transmitted human malaria. To this end he assembled a team of colleagues to make an all-out push. The team consisted of Dionisi who had worked with bird malaria and was to test Ross' findings; Bignami who would test his mosquito "bite theory"; Grassi, who knew the different kinds of mosquitoes, and who would survey the malarious and non-malarious areas and by comparing the mosquito populations try to deduce which species were possible transmitters, and Bignami together with Giovanni Bastianelli, a careful microscopist who knew his malaria parasites well, would follow Ross' trail to determine the parasite's development in the mosquito.

Since July 15, 1898, Grassi began to examine the marshes and swamps of Italy. Where Ross was patient and perseverant and willing to carry out a seemingly endless series of trial and error experiments. Grassi was methodical and analytical — he was also able to distinguish the different kinds of mosquitoes. Grassi observed "there was not a single place where there is malaria — where there aren't mosquitoes too, and either malaria is carried by one particular blood sucking mosquito out of the 40 different kinds of mosquitoes in Italy — or it isn't carried by mosquitoes at all."[8] Working in the Roman Campagna and the area surrounding it Grassi collected mosquitoes and at the same time recorded information on the incidence of malaria among the people. Soon it became apparent that most of the mosquitoes could be eliminated as carriers of the disease because they occurred where there was no malaria. There was, however, an exception. Where there were "zanzarone," as the Italians called the large brown, spotted winged mosquitoes, there was always malaria. Grassi recognized that the zanzarone were *Anopheles* and he wrote: "it is the anopheles mosquito that carries malaria ..." With this work Grassi was able to prove that "it is not the mosquito's children, but only the mosquito who herself bites a malaria sufferer — it is only that mosquito who can give malaria to healthy people." In September Grassi read a paper before the prestigious Accademia Nazionale dei Lincei in which he stated: "if mosquitoes do carry malaria, they are most certainly the zanzarone — *Anopheles* — not any of the 30–40 other species."[8]

Meanwhile the German government had dispatched Robert Koch, who previously had shown little interest in malaria, to German East Africa to solve the malaria problem. During his 1897–1898 sojourn in Tanganyika he claimed the natives of the Usambra Mountains called malaria "Mbu" because they thought the fever was carried by the Mbu, or the mosquito, which used to bite them as they moved into the lowlands. Upon his return to Germany in June 1898, Koch delivered a lecture at Berlin's Kaiserhof Hotel under imperial patronage with a band playing the national anthem in which he suggested that infected mosquitoes laid eggs on the human body, and afterwards malaria parasites emerged to enter the bloodstream. Koch was determined to solve the malaria puzzle by carrying out a research program in Italy, in particular in the Roman Campagna, where Grassi's own research was being carried out. Koch arrived triumphantly in August, visited Rome and its hospitals, and departed Italy in October having failed to solve the mystery of malaria transmission. Grassi was irritated by the way he and his colleagues had been virtually ignored when Koch "invaded" Italy presumably in order to grab the prize. Indeed, Koch meant to show that "only in the cloudy north was it possible for the star of science to shine for the illumination of the sleepy brains of the degenerate Italian race."[2] Grassi felt threatened by Koch, rushed to publish his findings, and to establish priority lest Koch claim to have solved the riddle for himself and Germany. In October 1898 Grassi announced that he and his colleagues were experimenting with *Culex* and *Anopheles* and expected a definitive solution to the question of transmission shortly. A month later *Culex* had been eliminated. In papers published in November and December Grassi and colleagues reported on the development of the parasite in *Anopheles*. Grassi infuriated Koch by sending him copies as a "Christmas present" and later declaring "the victory was completely ours."[2]

Grassi found that the development of human malaria in *Anopheles* was as had been predicted from Ross' studies of bird malaria. Grassi acknowledged the assistance of Bignami and Bastianelli but stated that the credit for the final completion belonged to him. Grassi also angered Ross with faint praise stating "it (the life cycle of *Plasmodium*) finds confirmation in that observed by Ross with the malaria of birds in the gray (*Culex*) mosquito."[2] Although the Italians attempted to place their work on an equal footing and parallel to Ross', the fact is they had a copy of his official report and had followed his published procedures step by step. Ross accused them of piracy.[9] Grassi, as egotistical and stubborn as Ross, fought back stating he had worked independent of Ross and had made his discoveries without any prior knowledge of what Ross had done. He stigmatized Ross' bird malaria research saying the figures and descriptions were incomprehensible, and he doubted whether they were of any value as a guide as to what happens in human malaria since similar parasites may have different life cycles. In 1902, Koch stood opposed to the Nobel committee since they were planning to split the prize for Physiology or Medicine between Ross and Grassi. Indeed, Grassi was considered by Koch to be an enemy, and he called him a charlatan with neither brains nor ethics. Ross alone received the Nobel Prize, but despite this award for "work on malaria, by which he has shown how it enters the organism and thereby has laid the foundation for successful research on this disease and methods of combating it," for the remainder of his life he was embittered. This was largely due to his easily taking offense and magnifying a petty slight out of all proportion. Even apologies from Bignami and Bastianelli and their dissociation from Grassi's increasingly arrogant contentions did not mollify Ross' contempt for the Italians.

Ross claimed that it was only after Grassi had read his work on the transmission of malaria using birds did he recognize that only in those areas where there was *Anopheles* was there human malaria, and that *Culex* was not involved, but Grassi did not publish this or the development of the parasite in these mosquitoes until late in 1898. Ross wrote in his *Memoirs*[9]: "they ... had this paper of mine before them when they wrote their note. Their statement was ... a deliberate and intentional lie, told in order to discredit my work and so to obtain priority ... Many of the items ... are directly pirated from my ... results ... stolen straight from me ..." For decades the arguments over priority and originality raged between Ross and Grassi. In truth, although Ross, based on his work with bird malaria, predicted that the parasite of human malaria must also be transmitted in a similar way it was Grassi and coworkers who actually conducted experiments on the transmission of human malaria, only they formulated and understood there was a closed cycle between mosquito and human, and it was the Italian school of malariologists including Grassi, Bignami and Bastianelli who were able to show the complete dependence on the *Anopheles* mosquito for transmission of human malaria.[11,12]

iv. A Hidden Life Revealed

Ronald Ross, shortly after discovering the mosquito as a vector for *Plasmodium*, presumed the inoculated sporozoites after entry into the blood stream burrowed straightaway into red blood cells. His rival Battista Grassi, however, suggested that the nucleus of the sporozoite was so different from that found in the blood stages that a considerable degree of transformation would be necessary to convert one directly into the other. Pursuing this line of thought, Grassi hypothesized in 1901 that an intermediate stage occurred somewhere in the body — a pre-blood (exo-erythrocytic or EE) form — and that this would carry out the necessary transformation. Grassi's hypothesis quickly fell apart when two years later Fritz Schaudinn (1871–1906), a preeminent microbe hunter, claimed the direct penetration of the red cell by the sporozoite. Schaudinn it is said took ripe and ruptured oocysts from a mosquito infected with *P. vivax*, placed it in a warmed, dilute drop of his own blood obtained from a blood blister he got from rowing and then peered through his microscope for six uninterrupted hours.[2] So persuasive was

Schaudinn's description — sporozoites pushed into the red cell, first making a dent, then penetrating with their pointed tail and lastly pulling themselves inside by peristaltic jerks — that even Grassi did not pursue the matter further. "Schaudinn's curious delusion lay like a spell over subsequent investigators" for decades.[2] However, "science is a study of errors slowly corrected" and soon indirect evidence questioned both the observations and conclusions of Schaudinn. First, there was the failure to confirm Schaudinn's microscopic findings and second in the treatment of patients with tertiary syphilis the effects of quinine were found to be markedly different in blood-induced infections from those that were sporozoite-induced. In this so called "therapy by malaria" the common practice was to induce malaria (mostly *P. vivax*) by direct inoculation of blood or by inoculating sporozoites by mosquito bite or in isolated salivary glands or in entire ground up mosquitoes. The blood-inoculated patients were cured with quinine whereas the sporozoite induced infections relapsed after the same quinine therapy. Even more telling were the observations of the American Clay Huff, the British Sydney Price James and the Australian Neil Fairley. During World War II, with the help of Australian army volunteers, Fairley measured the incubation period i.e. the time it took for parasites to appear in the blood after a mosquito-induced infection; in *P. vivax* it was eight days and in *P. falciparum* it was five days.[2] He also found that during the incubation period the blood was not infectious by transfusion (another overlooked clue was the case of Manson infecting his son with *P. vivax*-infected mosquitoes obtained from the Roman Campagna and where the parasites did not appear in the blood for 15 days). Malaria parasites must have been lurking somewhere in the body, but the question was where?

Beginning in the mid-1930s, Huff and Bloom and James and Tate and then others observed malaria parasites developing in endothelial cells and macrophages prior to the appearance of parasites in the red blood cells in bird as well as in lizard malarias. These pre-blood stages were called exo-erythrocytic, or EE, forms. Following Huff and Coulston's landmark description of the development of *P. gallinaceum* — from the entrance of sporozoites into the skin of chickens to the appearance of parasites in the blood — Huff boldly suggested: "since indirect evidence for ... exo-erythrocytic stages in mammalian malarias is good it would appear advisable to adopt their presence in sporozoite-induced infections as a working hypothesis ..."[13]

In 1945 Col. Sydney Price James told P. C. C. Garnham, then a young Medical Officer in Kenya, not to return from East Africa until he found pre-blood forms in mammalian malaria. James' gentle insistence proved stimulating to Garnham, and two years later, after James' death, in the Medical Research Laboratory, Nairobi, Garnham found EE stages in the liver of an African monkey infected with *P. kochi.*[14] Shortly thereafter Garnham joined H. E. Shortt at the London School of Tropical Medicine and Hygiene where work began using *P. cynomolgi* in rhesus monkeys with the expectation that the findings would relate to *P. vivax.* There were many attempts and many failures; success was finally achieved, however, when 500 infected mosquitoes were allowed to bite a single rhesus, then for good measure the infected mosquitoes were macerated in monkey serum, and this brew also injected. Seven days later the monkey was sacrificed and its organs taken for microscopic examination. Shortt expected that the EE stages would be found in locations similar to those described for bird malarias. This would turn out not to be the case. Instead, the site of pre-blood stages for *P. cynomolgi* was the liver, as had been the case with *P. kochi.* Shortt and Garnham promptly reported their findings in a paper published in *Nature.*[15] From that time forward pre-blood stages have been described for the non-human primate malarias,[16] the human malarias,[17–19] as well as in many of the rodent malarias.[20]

In *P. falciparum* infections, the disappearance of parasitized red cells from the peripheral circulation (as evidenced by simple microscopic examination of a stained blood film) may be followed by a reappearance of parasites in the blood. This type of relapse, called recrudescence, results from an increase in the number of pre-existing blood parasites. *P. vivax* and *P. ovale* also relapse, though the reappearance of parasites in the blood is not from a pre-existing population of blood stages and occurs after cure of the primary attack. The source of these blood stages remained controversial for many years but in 1980, the origin of such relapses was identified. In relapsing malarias, induced by sporozoites, Krotoski and coworkers found dormant parasites, called hypnozoites, within liver cells.[21] The hypnozoites, by an unknown mechanism, are able to initiate full EE development and then go on to establish a blood infection.

The pre-blood stages of monkeys and humans are difficult to study because of ethical considerations, the scarcity of suitable species of monkeys, the narrow range of human parasites adapted to primates, different pathologies in humans and primates, and because of expense. Humans are more plentiful, but the necessary numbers of volunteers willing to undergo liver biopsy are difficult to find. Moreover, even when a mosquito inoculates dozens of sporozoites into a human, and these successfully invade liver cells and develop into an EE form; only a few dozen may be present in a three-pound organ. It has been estimated if a mosquito inoculated 100 sporozoites there would be a single EE form found among a billion liver cells. Truly, the EE form is a needle in a haystack.

Today it is recognized that *Plasmodium* has three lives (Figure 1). Humans are infected through the bite of a female anopheline mosquito when

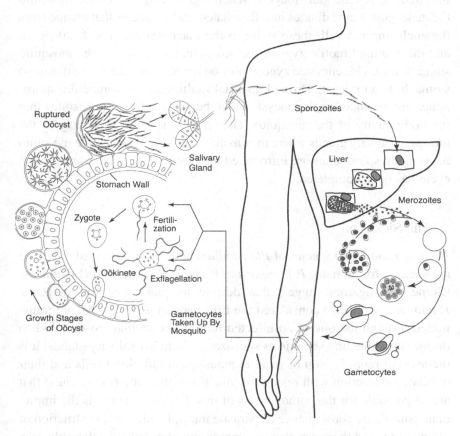

Figure 1.   The life cycle of the human malaria *P. falciparum*.

during blood feeding she injects sporozoites from her salivary glands. The inoculated sporozoites travel via the bloodstream to the liver where they enter liver cells. Within the liver cell the non-pigmented parasite, the pre-blood stage, multiplies asexually to produce 10,000 or more infective off-spring. These do not return to their spawning ground, the liver, but instead invade red blood cells (erythrocytes). By asexual reproduction of parasites in red blood cells (called erythrocytic schizogony or merogony) infectious offspring (merozoites) are released from erythrocytes. These can invade other red cells to continue the cycle of parasite multiplication, with extensive red blood cell destruction and deposition of hemozoin. In some cases the merozoites enter red cells but do not divide. Instead, they differentiate into male or female gametocytes. When ingested by the female mosquito the male gametocyte divides into flagellated microgametes that escape from the enclosing red cell, these swim to the macrogamete, one fertilizes it, and the resultant motile zygote, the ookinete, moves across the mosquito stomach wall. This encysted zygote, now on the outer surface of the mosquito stomach, is an oocyst. Through asexual multiplication, threadlike sporozoites are produced in the oocyst, which bursts to release sporozoites into the body cavity of the mosquito. The sporozoites find their way to the mosquito salivary glands where they mature, and when this female mosquito feeds again sporozoites are introduced into the body and the transmission cycle has been completed.

v. The Sickness

Although some 170 species of *Plasmodium* have been described only four are specific for humans, *P. falciparum*, *P. vivax*, *P. ovale*, and *P. malariae*. (Some investigators suggest that despite its preference for monkeys, *P. knowlesi* should be considered the fifth malaria parasite). All are transmitted through the bite of an infected female anopheline mosquito when during blood feeding she injects sporozoites from her salivary glands. It is the asexual reproduction of malaria parasites in red blood cells and their ultimate destruction with release of infectious offspring (merozoites) that are responsible for the pathogenesis of this disease. Anemia is the immediate pathologic consequence of parasite multiplication and destruction of erythrocytes and there can also be suppression of red blood cell production in the bone marrow. During the first few weeks of infection the spleen is palpable because it is swollen from the accumulation of parasitized red blood cells and the proliferation of white blood cells. At this time it is soft and easily ruptured. If the infection is treated the spleen returns to normal size; in chronic infections, however, the spleen continues to enlarge, becoming hard and blackened in color due to the accumulation of malaria pigment. The long-term consequences of malaria infections are an enlarged spleen and liver and organ dysfunction.[22]

The primary attack of malaria begins with headache, fever, anorexia, malaise, and aching muscles.[23] This is followed by paroxysms of chills, fever, and profuse sweating. The fever spike may reach up to 41°C and corresponds to the rupture of the red cell as merozoites are released from the infected cell. There may be nausea, vomiting, and diarrhea. Such symptoms are not unusual for an infectious disease and it is for this reason that malaria is frequently called "The Great Imitator." Then, depending on the species, the paroxysms tend to assume a characteristic periodicity. In *P. vivax, P. ovale,* and *P. falciparum* the periodicity is 48 hours; because the fevers recur every third day they are called "tertian malarias," while *P. malariae,* with its periodicity of 72 hours and fevers recurring every fourth day, is called "quartan malaria." *P. malariae* may persist in the body for up to four decades without signs of pathology. If the infection is not synchronous and there are several broods of parasites, the periodicity may occur at 24 hour intervals.

P. vivax which accounts for 45% of all malaria cases, results in severe and debilitating attacks but is rarely fatal, and hence it is called benign tertian malaria. It is able to remain in the body for a long period without reinfection, however, due to the persistence of "sleeping stages" (hypnozoites) in the liver. Indeed, *P. vivax* and *P. ovale* may remain in this state of suspended animation for three to five years before there is any sign of a blood infection. *P. malariae, P. ovale,* and *P. vivax* attack red blood cells of a particular age and hence do not cause severe anemia that may lead to death; *P. falciparum,* however, unlike the other three kinds is indiscriminate in its preference invading red blood cells of all ages, and as a result causes infections that are more severe and which untreated can result in a death rate of 25% in adults. Falciparum malaria is referred to as malignant tertian malaria to distinguish it from the other tertian malarias (*vivax* and *ovale*).

Complications of malaria include kidney insufficiency, kidney failure, fluid-filled lungs, neurological disturbances, and severe anemia. In the pregnant female falciparum malaria may result in stillbirth, lower than normal birth weight, or abortion. Non-immune persons and children may develop cerebral malaria, a consequence of the mechanical blockage of small blood vessels, and capillaries in the brain because of the sequestration of infected red blood cells. *P. falciparum* may either survive for a relatively short time in the body after causing an acute infection or it may kill, but most often it remains as a chronic infection. Falciparum malaria, occurring mostly in sub-Saharan Africa, accounts for 50% of all clinical malaria cases and is responsible for 95% of deaths.

Chapter 2

A Personal Scientific Odyssey

i. Early Years

I grew up in the city of New York. As a youngster in high school I took an advanced zoology course from Mrs. Marion Sweet and became fascinated by things biological. I drew pictures of the preserved specimens she brought into class and learned their diagnostic characteristics. I excelled in that course but for a while I entertained the idea that I might someday become a commercial artist. Thoughts of a career in art, however, were dashed when I took a drawing class as a high school senior; one day when I glanced across the aisle and saw the renderings by others in the class I found myself much less accomplished. Clearly, I recognized at an early age, art would not be a successful career path.

The City College of New York (CCNY), provided the opportunity of a higher education for those high school students who could pass the rigid requirements for entry. As was expected of me by my parents, and thanks to a good high school grade point average, I applied for and was admitted to CCNY. At the time of my entry CCNY had very high academic standards. And, it was affordable. Supported by public funds tuition was $6 per semester. (Today, 60 years later, the yearly tuition at CCNY is $6,030). There were also nominal fees for most science courses to cover the consumable costs of biology specimens (fetal pigs, lobsters, frogs, dogfish, cats) and breakage of laboratory glassware. We flattered ourselves by calling CCNY the poor man's Harvard. In fact, many of us, even if our parents could afford it (and mine couldn't) would have been unable to enroll as undergraduates at Harvard University since there was a quota for Jews. I decided to major in science and education with the goal of following in the footsteps of Mrs. Sweet to become a high school teacher. My poor grades in a freshman college chemistry class suggested that I was not cut out to be a teacher of that subject. I also had difficulty with calculus. But, with biology — taken in my sophomore year — it was different. In each and every biology class at CCNY, I received a grade of A. CCNY set a high bar for academic performance, however it was not a powerhouse in the doing of science. Most faculty members had heavy teaching loads and so there was neither the time nor the inclination towards research for most. As a result the majority of Biology faculty did not keep current in their field. Indeed during the time I was at CCNY I never heard about the role of the double helix of DNA, the structure of antibody or the nature of the immune system. There was no graduate program in Biology at CCNY, however a few Biology faculty did have appointments at the American Museum of Natural History and some engaged in graduate teaching at Columbia University. What characterized CCNY was an undergraduate body of smart and very aggressive students — slum kids, mostly Jews, whose immigrant parents wanted them to get a college education and in so doing be able to move out of the lower-middle class. I was an ambitious student attempting to master the material in the courses I took.

As a Biology student with exceptional grades at commencement I received the Ward Medal for Excellence in Biology. I stood out from the crowd (of high achievers) and was fortunate enough to become familiar on a one on one basis with some faculty members. Three in particular encouraged me to abandon my goal to be a high school science teacher (just like Mrs. Sweet) and to apply to graduate school. Thanks to William Tavolga (my instructor in Histology) and Herman Spieth (my instructor in Field Biology), both associated with the American Museum of Natural History, I was given an introduction to the eminent invertebrate zoologist, Libbie Hyman, at the Museum, and the Chair of the Department, the protozoologist, James Dawson, a friend of the Chair of Zoology at the University of Florida, W.C. Allee, arranged for my immediate acceptance to the University of Florida as well as a research assistantship at the University. The assistantship provided sufficient monies for graduate school tuition.

When I enrolled at the University of Florida in Gainesville it was my first time living outside of New York City, and it was an opportunity to do independent field research. I became a research assistant to Professor James Lackey in the Department of Sanitary Science. He asked me to sample the waters in the Gulf of Mexico (presumably to look at pollution) and to characterize the one-celled animals (*protozoa*) I saw. To identify what I saw under the microscope he gave me a dichotomous key written in German (*Die Tierwelt Deutschlands*) by Alfred Kahl. I spent long hours peering through the microscope, worked diligently translating German into English, and had some measure of success in protozoan identification and possibly even discovered a new species. I wrote a report on my find- ings suggesting avenues for further study. I also excelled in the graduate courses — Embryology, Advanced Invertebrate Zoology, Biological Literature and Institutions — I took. But my time in Florida was abbrevi- ated to one semester when I received notice that I was to be drafted into the U.S. Army. The reasoning of the Selective Service Board was that there was a draft on, and I had college deferments during my years at CCNY — the time of the Korean War. Now it was time to do my duty. Despite my academic success at the University of Florida I was not unhappy to leave the deeply segregated environment of Florida, and I was less than satisfied that the Department of Zoology had as its emphasis herpetology and ichthyology rather than protozoology. Further, the Zoology faculty members (aside from Allee) were (at least to my mind) an undistinguished lot.

In August of 1954, I was inducted into the U.S. Army. I did infantry basic training at Ft. Dix, and hoped to stay out of combat by training as a Medical Laboratory Technician at Ft. Sam Houston in Texas, however this was not to be since the school for training Medical Laboratory Technicians was no longer operating. Instead I was trained as a Medical Technician (Med Tech) — essentially an aide to a nurse — at Ft. Sam Houston and then at Valley Forge Army Hospital in Phoenixville, PA. Upon completion of Med Tech training I was shipped overseas to a Medical Clearing Company at Camp Roeder in Salzburg, Austria. Despite many months of training to be a nurses' aide a sergeant told me that I would become a truck driver. However, I was saved from this fate by claiming poor eyesight and an ability to do laboratory work. Thus, through pure serendipity and chutzpah, as well as on-the-job training I became a Medical Laboratory Technician (Lab Tech) doing bacteriology, hematology, parasitology, venipuncture, immunizations, and the like. This laboratory experience lasted three months and when the Austrian Command was closed I was shipped to the 7th Evacuation Hospital in Darmstadt, Germany. By this time the Korean War had ended and there was no war in Europe so there were no wounded bodies to clear or evacuate; most days were spent in classes or in field exercises — mainly erecting tents for the evacuation hospital and its related facilities. I volunteered to work in the Medical Laboratory of the Dispensary of the Hospital and did this for nine months and also spent three months in Heidelberg, Germany (at the 101st Station Hospital) doing similar work. The laboratory experiences in Austria and Germany focused my attention on disease — there was an abundance of venereal disease among the soldiers, worm infections in the food handlers, and clinical cases of blood disorders in the dependents. It wasn't what one would call real science and it certainly wasn't scientific research, but I did learn to handle syringes, pipettes, test tubes, was able to run routine clinical tests and I did not shirk from dealing with samples of blood, urine, and feces. After two years in the Army I returned to civilian life, and although I had not been completely satisfied with my graduate life at the University of Florida, I decided that in my time in Europe I had matured sufficiently to be able to adapt to life in the American South. Further, I was offered a University Fellowship with full tuition and a stipend. After six weeks of graduate study at the University of Florida, however, I found myself wanting. I wanted better professors and courses, and a more challenging research program. I met with Professor Lackey and told him of my disappointment with the didactic training and that I was planning to leave graduate school. He tried to convince me that I could do more research and spend less time in the courses. I indicated that that would not do. He asked, "When do you intend to leave?" "Tonight," I replied. "Then," he said, "there is no sense in further discussion." I'm sure he regarded me as immature and impetuous. And for a while, after my return to New York, and when I couldn't find any work in research and had to teach 7th and 8th grade Math and Science in Public School 5 (in Yonkers, NY) I agreed with Professor Lackey's assessment. Successful as I was as a Junior High School teacher I was convinced that this was not what I wanted to do for the rest of my life. I decided despite this interruption in graduate study I would not give up on my goal of becoming a research scientist.

During the time I was 'lost' in Yonkers I sought academic refuge at CCNY. I was hired to teach in the Introductory Biology classes in the Evening Division at CCNY with a very gifted teacher, Alexander Chaikelis (1901–1981), who (like myself) received his B.S. from CCNY (1926). Although he received a Ph.D. from Columbia University (1933) he did not do research after joining the CCNY faculty. He did however serve as my mentor for teaching Biology at the college level. I also took graduate courses in Genetics, and in the Biological Foundations of Animal Behavior. This latter course was with William Etkin (1906–1999).

Etkin too had a B.S. from CCNY (1928). He followed this with a Ph.D. from the University of Chicago in 1934 and shortly thereafter joined the CCNY faculty; he had a joint appointment with the Albert Einstein School of Medicine and was an endocrinologist, evolutionist and an expert on metamorphosis and animal behavior. He taught the undergraduate course in Vertebrate Anatomy, but was ham handed and when asked for help with a dissection he ripped through most tissues eventually finding the desired anatomical part but in the process destroying everything else. He then announced in a stentorian voice "There she stands in all her naked beauty." Etkin was one of those fabled teachers who could inspire and weave knowledge, learning, and research into a fascinating fabric. I didn't have any undergraduate courses with him however I did seek his advice when I took his course on the Biological Basis of Social Behavior. I told Etkin that I was thinking of taking a position as a research technician. He counseled me that with only a B.S. degree there was little likelihood I'd ever become an independent researcher. He replied, "If you really want to do laboratory research, and run with the hounds, get thee to graduate school on a full-time basis, and a doctorate." It was sage advice.

In 1957, I received a CCNY Biology Club Scholarship three years after graduation! (This was due to the efforts of Roslyn Moskowitz, the Department of Biology secretary, a spinster who had an exceptional fondness for me). I took the Scholarship money to enroll in the Invertebrate Zoology course at the Marine Biological Laboratory (MBL) in Woods Hole, MA. There I discovered what biology was all about. At the MBL I was able to spend all day, every day, for six weeks studying live invertebrates. The field trips were extraordinary, especially for a South Bronx slum kid, and the faculty were exceptional: Clark Read (Johns Hopkins), Howard Schneiderman (Cornell), John Buck (NIH), Theodore Bullock (UCLA), Grover Stephens (Minnesota), Morris Rockstein (NYU), John Anderson (Cornell), and Cadet Hand (Berkeley). During that summer the faculty recognized me as a promising student (and I did rediscover an oval window on the 5th walking leg of the lobster). At summer's end I was invited to be the lab assistant for the Invertebrate Zoology course for the next two summers; I readily accepted and shared the work with another young parasitologist, Frank Friedl, from the University of Minnesota.

I was lucky to have grown up in New York City where in the public education system there were dedicated teachers who set high academic standards and where one was judged on performance rather than on race, religion, background, income or concepts of self-esteem. CCNY offered those of us with brainpower but without money or influential connections to compete with and often surpass graduates of the most prestigious Ivy League schools. CCNY equipped me to write, think and communicate effectively and it was fierce competition that so sharpened the intellect that some of us were able to succeed when matched against the best and brightest from other highly regarded academic institutions. At CCNY I was fortunate to have mentors — Professors — who really cared about my future, who were there to provide guidance and who were instrumental in my obtaining support for graduate study.

ii. Graduate Studies

Having experienced graduate study at the University of Florida and the effects of racial segregation I decided to avoid all graduate schools south of the Mason–Dixon Line. To find the 'best' grad school for my interest in parasites I scoured University catalogs for those offering the greatest number of courses in parasitology. Eventually I settled on Northwestern University (or more accurately, they settled on me). I was awarded an Abbott Laboratory Fellowship with a young Assistant Professor, Robert Hull. After serving in the U.S. Army, he received a B.S. (Chemistry 1949), M.S. (1950) and as a graduate student of the eminent protozoologist

R.R. Kudo, a Ph.D. (Zoology, Biochemistry, Physiology 1953) at the University of Illinois. His doctoral work was on an unusual group of predatory ciliates, the suctoria. At the time of my arrival at Northwestern University (1957) Hull's lab was also carrying out malaria research using the bird malaria, *Plasmodium lophurae*. Hull was tall and lean, had a serious demeanor most of the time and was a chain smoker. For some of us he acted in a fatherly fashion. He became a confidante, invited us to his home for holidays and when I needed an automobile to get from my apartment to the lab, he went with me to the dealership, kicked the tires of a used car, and advised me to purchase a 1955 Pontiac. His interests in protozoa and parasites were broad; the laboratory had parasites growing in chickens (*P. lophurae*), bees, (*Nosema apis*) snakes (*Macdonaldius seetae*), a variety of laboratory grown protozoa (*Tetrahymena* and *Paramecium*) as well as suctoria recovered from Lake Michigan and us — his graduate students. Each graduate student occupied a desk in the lab that adjoined his office. He gave unstintingly of his time and was always on call. This seemingly limitless interest in all things microscopic coupled with his obvious lack of personal experience with such diverse groups of protozoans turned out to be a handicap to some of his students. Indeed, it was accepted by myself that the research inexperienced Hull would be unable to provide the guidance necessary for a doctoral thesis. In short, my thesis research would develop independently or not at all. Hull did putter around the lab fixing instruments and trying to get a Cartesian diver apparatus working in order to measure the oxygen consumption of a single suctorian during feeding, and twice a week he inoculated a fresh batch of chickens with blood taken from malaria-infected chickens.

Hull's first graduate student working on malaria was a Vietnamese priest, Father Hoang Quoc Truong. Truong (whose research aside from his 1956 Ph.D. thesis was never published) found that as the chickens aged they became increasingly resistant to a bird malaria (*P. lophurae)* infection, and after one-month of age chickens were able to survive a level of infection as high as 70–80%, a level that invariably killed younger birds. He observed resistance to re-infection by the older birds and was able to reduce the severity of the infection by transfusion of plasma from either recovered or older chicks. This reduction of the infection (that is, immunity), was dependent on the amount of "immune" plasma transfused into the recipient birds, had already been demonstrated with another bird malaria, *P. circumflexum*[24]; however, they felt "that whatever immune substances are present in serum must be there in relatively small concentration." Father Truong went a step further showing the immune substance could also be demonstrated by incubation of parasitized red cells for one hour with "immune" plasma, and he showed that "immune" activity was associated with the globulin fraction. Truong's work was not entirely novel. Indeed, in the early 1950s Lucy and William Hay Taliaferro (who were on the faculty of the University of Chicago just a few miles south of Northwestern University) found evidence of acquired immunity in both *P. gallinaceum* and *P. lophurae*; it appeared progressively in the former and suddenly at the peak of infection in the latter. Immunity to re-infection resulted mainly from parasite-killing (parasiticidal) antibodies in both species, which acted on both free merozoites and the parasites within the red cell. Indeed, 97–99% of the re-infecting parasites were destroyed within 36 hours, whereas parasite reproduction was only temporarily decreased. The reproduction-inhibiting effects were not apparent when the re-infecting dose was large enough to break down the acquired immunity that they ascribed to parasite-killing antibodies. Their conclusion: after the acquisition of immunity, the few surviving parasites of each brood are apparently resistant to both parasite-killing and reproduction-inhibiting mechanisms.

My own studies of malaria immunity and vaccines began with *P. lophurae* infections in white Leghorn chickens that had been established by Father Truong (who upon completion of his thesis research returned to Vietnam and so we never met). As Hull's research assistant, I was put to work on the NIH supported malaria project, however I had no clue what I should do. Hull was of little help. He provided me with almost no advice save for indicating the coursework I should take: introductory Parasitology/ Protozoology — courses he taught — as well as Experimental Embryology (with Ray Watterson, 1915–1984), Experimental Cytology (with Robert C. King, b. 1928) and Invertebrate Zoology (with Frank Brown 1908–1983). To bolster my biochemical background I was to take Biochemistry and Physical Chemistry. When I heard him mentioning these two latter courses I panicked. I had only a summer course in Organic Chemistry and was not strong in the Inorganic Chemistry and Calculus courses taken at CCNY. I sought the counsel of Irving M. Klotz (1916–2005) who was one of the leading thinkers of his time in physical bio-chemistry, the field connecting physical chemistry with the life sciences, and an expert on protein structure. He encouraged me to enroll in these courses telling me to apply myself. He went further saying the courses would stand me in good stead — this was the direction modern biology was going. Klotz became one of my mentors and allowed his analytical ultracentrifuge — a behemoth of a machine costing many tens of thou-sands of dollars and the only one in the Chemistry Department — be made available to me for my thesis research. I did well in all the graduate courses taken at Northwestern University including Physical Chemistry and Biochemistry (with Lazlo Lorand, an expert on proteases and an émigré from Hungary who later became a friend during summers in Woods Hole). Persistence paid off.

King was interested in developmental genetics and had isolated a large number of female-sterile mutations in the fruit fly *Drosophila* and I was able to study one of these (an eye mutant named morula). Years later when I was a post-doctoral at the Rockefeller Institute (see p. 37) dining in Welch Hall I met the 78-year-old Clara Lynch (1882–1985) who first described the relationship of sterility to this mutant in the Columbia University laboratory of T. H. Morgan and Calvin Bridges. When I asked her whether her work in the legendary Fly Room at Columbia with these pioneers in *Drosophila* genetics was more exciting than today she said "No, it's much more exciting today." She was forever young and a delight to know! I hoped as I matured as a scientist I could be more like her.

To find a topic worthy of a research thesis I spent many months in the library reading research articles and taking notes from the abstracts in the *Tropical Disease Bulletin*, read the *Journal of Infectious Diseases*, the *Journal of Hygiene* and Hewitt's 1940 treatise *Bird Malaria*. These notes I kept in a bound book. I then spent many more months reading blood films from infected chickens that I had treated with various immune-blocking agents such as trypan blue and carbon ink. All I got from this work were chickens with black and blue colored spleens and livers! On my own, I decided to see whether the immunity developed in chickens was strong. I was able to inject recovered chickens with large volumes of infected blood and by the time I was able to make the first blood smear there wasn't a single infected red cell to be seen on the slide. What, I wondered, was the basis of this immunity?

At Northwestern University carrying out research was up to the efforts of the individual. There was no hand holding. Hull felt that performing routine lab chores such as washing glassware and preparation of media as well as caring for our animals was as essential to graduate training as was critical thinking and skill in laboratory procedures. Of course, it also meant that he didn't have to provide a salary for a dishwasher or an animal caretaker. In a dank, dark, smelly animal room in the basement of Locy Hall the chicks were held in cages called battery brooders. Each cage was fitted with a tray holding water and another tray was filled with chicken feed. Lacking an animal caretaker it was my job to replenish the food, clean out the food debris from the water trays, refill the trays with clean water and replace the newspaper in the trays that held the chicken feces. On the occasion Hull also pitched in feeding, watering, and cleaning of the cages and he passaged the infection. These were, I believe, chores he liked doing and in his mind probably justified his being a contributor to the research. In a humorous situation, he assisted in the capture of a runaway chicken. It must have been quite a sight to see the two of us, butterfly nets in hand, running around the parking lot trying to retrieve a chicken that had flown out of a garbage can when I had not completely euthanized it. Whether by accident or design Hull found greater reward in his various administrative duties in the Society of Protozoologists, Sigma Xi, and in talking about research rather than doing it. I had one embarrassing experience when Hull was trying to impress James Moulder (1921–2011) a distinguished microbiologist and a member of Taliaferro's department at the University of Chicago. Hull fabricated a story about the research I was doing. After telling the tall tale he turned to me and said, "Isn't that right Irwin?" I was struck silent. From that time forward I lost respect for him, his lack of integrity, and for his attempt to compromise mine. Valuable lessons I learned from the time I spent in the Hull laboratory were: be independent, choose your mentors carefully, do not conceal your blunders even if it might turn out to be embarrassing, be persistent, read the literature, and to become a respected and productive scientist shun administrative responsibilities.

In 1963, Hull moved to Florida State University to become the Chairman and Professor of Biological Sciences. In 1968–1969, he was elected President of the Society of Protozoologists. Regrettably, his heavy smoking (especially Kent cigarettes with the micronite filter) caught up with him and he died from cancer on July 13, 1970. It was a tradition of the Society to have the Presidential address at its annual luncheon. I was called by Bronislaw Honigberg an officer of the Society and asked 'as Hull's most famous student' could I deliver a eulogy in lieu of the Presidential address? I was conflicted. Should I describe Hull warts and all or would it be more appropriate to gild the lily? I opted for the latter, convincing myself that by emphasizing the positive in his life little harm would be done. Addressing the assembled members I became choked with emotion as I read the eulogy I had written. When I left the podium one of Hull's graduate students who was a contemporary of mine (Richard Albach, 1931–2010, then a Professor at the Chicago Medical School) said to me "If I didn't know better even I might have been convinced by your crocodile tears." The eulogy was published in the 1971 issue of the *Journal of Protozoology*.

Graduate school life at Northwestern University was, unlike CCNY, idyllic. Evanston was a "dry town" whose tree-lined avenues were filled with well-manicured lawns and elegant homes. In order to have any alcoholic beverages one had to cross the line from Evanston into Chicago. There was virtually no crime in affluent Evanston, and the streets were safe both day and night. There were no tenements. The campus itself was beautiful, bordered Lake Michigan and had rooming houses for graduate students. During my first year I lived in, of all places, Sherman House. It was within walking distance of the Biology Department and in subsequent years I shared an apartment with several other graduate students a few miles from campus. By auto it took only 10 minutes to drive from home to campus. The faculty in the Department of Biology, numbering at the time approximately a dozen, was by and large not outstanding researchers although there were a few 'stars.' Well-recognized in their field were Orlando Park in ecology, Robert C. King in genetics/cytology, Frank A. Brown Jr. in invertebrate zoology/biological rhythms, Maurice Sussman a microbiologist working on development in slime molds and Lewis H. Tiffany in nonvascular botany. Ray Watterson was an excellent embryologist and a superb teacher. Watterson was a warm and decent person but not a prolific researcher. In his Experimental Embryology class we were able to transplant chick limb buds, and pieces of epidermis and ablate certain tissues to determine their effects on development. These were exciting times in the graduate laboratory. I never had such hands on lab experiences at CCNY or at the University of Florida.

Graduate students were required to take classes and pass them with not less than a C grade. We also had to spend time as a teaching assistant, had to pass written and oral qualifying exams for the Ph.D. (The M.S. did not require a thesis but could be completed by two years of coursework). Passing the oral qualifying exam administered by a committee of 3–5 professors was a terrifying hurdle. Using what leadership skills I possessed I helped organize the other grad students so that after each had been through the oral qualifying exam they were debriefed. The questions and answers and by whom they were posed became a part of a written record that could be accessed by any grad student. A similar sharing of information followed the written exams. I received a non-thesis M.S. in two years, passed the qualifying exams, and completed the research for a Ph.D. a year later.

The Department of Biology at Northwestern University was housed in a three story concrete building, Cresap Laboratory. In the Hull laboratory the facilities were far from lavish. There was no fancy or high-powered apparatus for doing biochemical research. It had the usual array of glassware, a fraction collector, Klett colorimeter, Beckman DU spectrophotometer, a refrigerated centrifuge, an assortment of power supplies, refrigerators, deep freezer, microscopes, and incubators. What was not available was borrowed. Studying the blood stages of malaria microscopically I was fascinated by the deposition of the golden-brown–black malaria pigment called hemozoin. Believing it to be involved in immunity I decided to do a physicochemical characterization of the pigment using Klotz's ultracentrifuge, advice from Lorand on solubilization and to characterize the solutions by spectrophotometery. (The project was not entirely original; hemozoin had been analyzed in other laboratories, especially in the UK, and there was little evidence for it playing a role in immunity). I analyzed the pigment and found it to contain heme and to be coupled to a protein. Self-taught in immunology I used paper electrophoresis — then a relatively new biochemical method — to separate the serum components and found that the γ-globulin increased in amount by the fourth day, decreased to its original value by day seven, and that during this period there was a change in its mobility in the electric field. Further, a rise in the β-globulin on the 4th day persisted into the latent period, suggesting the presence of anti-parasite antibodies in this fraction. I found no evidence for hemozoin being a factor in inducing immunity. In fact, due to its poor solubility it appeared to be inert.

My doctoral thesis was a hodge-podge of self-directed malaria research, much of it lacking in imagination. But, it was sufficient to garner me a Ph.D. (1960). Knowing that I didn't have sufficient training to become a practicing research scientist I sought to further my experience. In short, I needed to find a post-doctoral position.

iii. The Rockefeller Institute and Post-doctoral Research

The winter before I completed my Ph.D. I spent the Christmas holidays in New York City visiting with my parents. During that time I dropped in to see Frank Friedl, with whom I had shared the Invertebrate Zoology lab assistant duties at the MBL. Frank had finished his Ph.D. and was now a post-doctoral fellow at the Rockefeller Institute working in the laboratory of the distinguished helminthologist Norman R. Stoll, author of among many papers, "This Wormy World." Frank suggested that I stop in and see William Trager on the third floor of Theobald Smith Hall, just across from Stoll's labs. Trager was the "dean" of malaria researchers. I had no appointment, but Friedl insisted Trager would not mind meeting me. When I entered, Trager was seated at his desk at the far end of his office. I expected (based on reputation) that he would be a tall and distinguished gentleman. However, when he rose to greet me, he stood no more than five feet two inches. He was slim, had thinning wavy brown hair, and wore wire rim glasses, a tie and a white shirt with sleeves rolled up. When he spoke his voice was almost squeaky. It was a disarming first encounter. We chatted in a very relaxed manner; he graciously listened to my account of what I was doing. At the end of our meeting it was clear (to me) that if I wanted to be a post-doctoral fellow in his laboratory I would receive his support.

It wasn't hard to leave Northwestern for Rockefeller. Northwestern University was not a bastion of science and Hull was not (at least in my eyes) a well-respected microbe hunter. After meeting with Trager, where I felt the prospective move to Rockefeller had already been sealed, I did the politic thing to try to make Hull feel that he had been instrumental in my obtaining the post-doctoral position. I asked him to please contact Trager and to endorse my coming to Rockefeller. He did so, and Hull was left with the impression that his recommendation had been the critical factor. This accidental meeting at the Rockefeller Institute affected my scientific career for the next 40 years, when Trager offered me a place in his laboratory at the Institute — where Paul de Kruif (author of *Microbe Hunters*) called it a 'shrine of science.' In the summer of 1960 my parents fearful of flying traveled by train from New York City to Chicago to attend commencement exercises at Northwestern University where I received the Ph.D. They were thrilled and convinced they actually saw me on the stage as I received the degree with hundreds of others. Afterwards they returned to New York City by train and I drove my 1955 Pontiac arriving two days later to move in with my parents at 1056 Boynton Avenue in the South Bronx. I returned home to begin my training in malaria research!

In late 1959 Trager and I corresponded regarding my application for an NIH Post-doctoral Fellowship and his submission of a research grant application to the NIH in support of the research on immunity I proposed to carry out at Rockefeller. On January 15, 1960 I received word that I was awarded a Research Fellowship Award (EF011, 320) with a stipend of $4,500 and $49 for travel beginning July 1, 1960 (provided I completed the requirements for the Ph.D.). The NIH awarded 'Associate Professor Dr. William Trager' and I a research grant (E-3550) for three years beginning September 1, 1960. The first year amount was $8,980 and somewhat less for subsequent years. The title of the project was: biochemical changes accompanying malarial infection. On June 1 I received a letter from Douglas Whitaker, the Vice President for Administration, stating that "President Detlev W. Bronk authorizes me to inform you that you are appointed Guest Investigator in the Rockefeller Institute ... July 1, 1960." (Being a Guest Investigator meant the Rockefeller Institute would not have to pay me a salary.)

Since I had an automobile (the 1955 Pontiac which I parked on the street near my parents' apartment house) I could drive to the Rockefeller Institute, with its free parking, or ride the subway in inclement weather. On July 1 I took the IRT subway from home in the Bronx to 68th Street and Lexington Avenue in Manhattan and walked from there to 66th Street and York Avenue — the entrance to the Rockefeller Institute.

The Institute had its origins in the early 1900s when John D. Rockefeller Sr. had his first grandson die of scarlet fever at age three. Rockefeller had made millions as a robber baron in the oil business and upon retirement from his position as head of Standard Oil devoted his life to philanthropy. Upon the advice of Frederick T. Gates Rockefeller pledged $200,000 to establish the Rockefeller Institute for Medical Research in 1901. The Institute gave grants and conducted research in makeshift quarters at 50th Street and Lexington Avenue. An outbreak of meningitis in 1904–1905 led the Institute's first Director, Simon Flexner to develop an antiserum for the disease. Rockefeller purchased a riverfront parcel from 64th Street to 67th Street and in later years expanded north and south. The first building, Founders Hall, opened in 1906 at the foot of 66th Street, followed in 1910 by a hospital and other buildings. The Department of Animal Pathology of the Institute was in Princeton, NJ and from 1915–1929 its Director was Theobald Smith (1859–1934). The Department (including Trager who joined the department in 1934) moved to New York City in 1947 and the New Jersey site was permanently closed in 1950.

The Rockefeller Institute was a place where the members were offered the opportunity to do full time research without the distractions of teaching or clinical work. There were autonomous departments headed by handpicked scientists selected with regard only to their prior achievements and interests in medical research. The Institute's 14-acre campus perched high above the East River has panoramic views of it and the borough of Queens. Looking up from FDR Drive one sees a massive craggy retaining wall resembling a castle fortification — the Rockefeller Institute. Buildings named Founders, Welch, Flexner, Smith, an animal house, and a President's residence are set back from the city proper behind a tall fence and planted grounds from what is now York Avenue. In the 1950s the distinctive Caspary Auditorium, a domed lecture hall was built, as was

Abbey Aldrich with living quarters for guests, an elegant dining room and by that time to accommodate the initiation of graduate programs graduate student housing.

As I walked up the drive at the front of 66th Street and climbed the steps to enter the foyer of Founders Hall I was greeted by a stone bust of John D. Rockefeller Sr. looking much like a wrinkled old prune. Further along was Welch Hall (built in 1929) that served as the Institute's library and also housed (until 1971) the Members dining facility. My initial reaction was one of awe. Walking these halls I remembered reading Sinclair Lewis' medical novel *Arrowsmith* and Paul de Kruif's *Microbe Hunters*. Both had an association with the Institute. De Kruif had been hired by Flexner in 1920 after he had received his Ph.D. from the University of Michigan in 1916 with Frederick G. Novy, who in turn had trained with Robert Koch in Germany and Emile Roux in Paris at the Pasteur Institute. Novy was a scientist of rigorous principles and a demanding mentor to de Kruif. In Novy's lab de Kruif worked on anaphylaxatoxin from dead trypanosomes. At the Rockefeller he worked on 'bacterial dissociation' — a change in phenotype — de Kruif realized was due to a gene mutation however at the time bacterial genetics was in its infancy and his explanations for the phenomenon, went largely unappreciated. (Indeed, had de Kruif remained he might have discovered that the transforming principle was DNA). In 1922 de Kruif was forced to resign from the Institute after he anonymously published a four-part polemic in *Century Magazine* about the conflict between science, commercialism, and charlatanism in medicine. The articles mocked the Institute's research objectives, purposes, methods, and organization. When President Flexner, who considered the promotion of team spirit as crucial to the ethos of the Institute, discovered that de Kruif was not only the author of the articles, he had used insider information and in so doing violated the rules, he strongly advised de Kruif to resign. Even de Kruif's mentor at the Institute, the eminent physiologist, Jacques Loeb, and a good friend could not or would not intervene because as he said 'powerful influences' were 'determined to get' de Kruif's 'scalp.' De Kruif who had been thinking of swapping his life as a medical researcher for that of a writer resigned. De Kruif then assisted and provided crucial scientific elements to Sinclair Lewis in the writing of *Arrowsmith*. The medical novel was initially to be a genuine co-production

with both being given authorship however the publisher looking to capital-
ize on the fame of Lewis insisted that the book bear only Lewis' name as
author. The book, published in 1925, was a best seller and with its publication the friendship between the two was shattered.

In 1923, after de Kruif finished with his work with Lewis on
Arrowsmith he took up residence in London and began research for his
first independent book, *Microbe Hunters*. His small circle of friends
helped de Kruif with his collection of 12 biosketches of the medical
researchers or doctors who had carried out major experiments. The book
showed their endurance and sacrifices as well as their breakthroughs and
small-mindedness. The personalities became real and the stories fascinating when he put words in the mouths of certain microbe hunters that they
never spoke. De Kruif's flamboyant and romantic style of writing contributed to the overwhelming success of *Microbe Hunters* and it captured the
imagination of an entire generation of young scientists (such as myself)
who were interested in becoming the new conquerors of disease.

Now 40 years later I was following in the footsteps of de Kruif (hop-
ing of course not to suffer the same fate). I was entering the Rockefeller
Institute and it was as Lewis described it in *Arrowsmith* as the fictional
McGurk Institute: a place that was to offer optimal conditions for research.
Free of economic constraints where world famous scientists would conduct their investigations in sophisticated ambience. Equipped with excellent infrastructure, and the best and latest devices, working autonomously
without interference, and provided with everything for their research. The
Institute's Welch dining hall where inspiring conversation, it was hoped,
would promote team spirit linked the laboratories socially. Here one
would be able to rub shoulders with the world's medical great. At lunch in
Welch Hall (de Kruif disparagingly described it as 'a scientific beanery')
one could talk with the scientific elite, a bevy of biological/immunological/
biochemical big names. What I would find during my time at Rockefeller
was that some of the Members would have their vanities, some would be
full of self-admiration and some could be petty. There was little in the way
of team spirit and in some instances competition led to backbiting. Some
Members rested on their laurels and did little research. Some would be
compromised by economic constraints and some exceptionally gifted
scientists could (and did) serve as role models for me.

The overriding themes in *Arrowsmith* are the role of science in society, the inevitable conflict between career and personal life, the in-fighting at academic and research institutions and the taint that comes from the over-commercialization in the discovery process. These would be themes that I would grapple with as I matured as a research scientist, but for the time being I was off to the Trager laboratory.

William Trager (1910–2005) received a doctorate from Harvard University in 1933. He spent his entire career at Rockefeller, although he lived at different times in Panama and Nigeria to do research. His research career began with insect cultivation and he developed the first bacteria-free culture system for mosquito larvae. His doctoral research under L. R. Cleveland at Harvard was on the intestinal termite flagellates that digest the cellulose in the wood eaten by the termite. In 1933 he became a Fellow of the National Research Council at the Rockefeller Institute's Department of Animal and Plant Pathology, and became a staff member in 1934. In 1939, Trager discovered acquired immunity to ixodid ticks. He also found ways to grow the tissues of tsetse flies, mosquitoes, and silk-worms so that sleeping sickness, encephalitis, and other diseases the insects carried could be studied. In World War II, as a Captain in the Sanitary Corps, he was sent to northern Australia and New Guinea to oversee the trials of a new antimalarial drug, atabrine, to see if it would help troops in the Pacific suffering from repeated malaria infections. After the war he returned to the Institute in Princeton, to begin work on malaria. From 1943–1947 he was able to show that biotin and a fat-soluble factor influenced chick susceptibility to *P. lophurae*. And shades of Father Truong and my own doctoral research he found that the globulin fraction from adult chickens, when injected into young chicks and ducklings, less-ened the number of parasites in the blood indicating that adult chicken plasma contained immune factors. In 1950, the Department of Animal and Plant Pathology (including Trager) moved to the Rockefeller Institute for Medical Research in New York City and there he began to pursue system-atic studies on the conditions promoting the survival and development of malaria parasites.

Trager used to say that 'you can't study something you can't grow.' He was always interested in growing things. He believed that if you under-stood the nutritional needs of a parasite you would be able to understand the molecular basis of parasitism. His approach was: once you got a culture established you could start removing bits from it and in the process discover what is crucial in the medium for that parasite. Rockefeller had lavish facilities, endless apparatus specially made in a wonderful machine shop, and technical know-how. Unlike Northwestern University, lab servants washed the glassware and cooked the media. Trager had two laboratories and an adjoining office. Each laboratory had a laboratory technician who could do the experiments for you and a dishwasher to wash the test tubes and assorted glassware. I was to occupy one of the labs with another post-doctoral, Philip D'Alesandro, and we would share a laboratory technician (Theresa Caporossi) and a Hungarian refuge was our dishwasher (Mary Sokoyi). Since there was only one desk in the post-doctoral lab and that was already occupied by D'Alesandro my 'desk' was at a longish table just to the right of Trager's desk in his office. His (or should I say our) office had no computer, and no typewriter but it did have a telephone.

Trager was meticulous about his daily routine. Each morning he would travel by train from Scarsdale to Grand Central Station and walk from 42nd Street to his Rockefeller lab on 68th Street and York Avenue. Arriving he would first stop at the office remove his coat, jacket and tie and place them in the closet, roll up his sleeves and then move into the lab sometimes wearing a white lab coat. In his lab he prepared the reagents weighing out the various ingredients using a Sartorius analytical balance or a top loading Mettler balance. He then placed the dry medium in a flask, added water, the flask opening was plugged with cotton and he had the technician send it down to the media room to be sterilized. For use in culture he assembled his equipment — a Bunsen burner, plugged pipettes, medium, slides, culture dishes under the glass framed Theobald Smith hood and proceeded to transfer medium into the dishes with impeccable sterile technique. He never added antibiotics to his media. When samples were to be taken he again used sterile technique, flaming his instruments in the Bunsen burner flame, taking samples to make thin blood films and then these were given to his technician for staining. He used phase contrast or light microscopy to read the slides. At day's end (with a break for lunch in Welch Hall where he had to shed his lab coat and put on a tie and jacket) he recorded the results of an experiment in a bound notebook in his scrawly barely legible handwriting. He would leave at exactly 4:45 p.m. to catch a train from Grand Central Station to home. Once, while we were deep into discussion, he looked at his pocket watch, stood up, put on his overcoat, and left the office. I was so engrossed in my description of the lab results that I followed him out, we walked quickly to Grand Central talking all the way right up to the train. When the door of the train opened, Trager got in and said, "See you tomorrow" leaving me on the platform somewhat speechless.

Trager, having no teaching responsibilities, was a fully engaged bench scientist. Indeed, I regarded him as a scientist's scientist. He was a specialist in the nutrition of blood protozoa — especially malaria and hemoflagellates — and he rarely ventured out of this domain. He did little work in immunology although early in his career he tried to blockade the immune system with carbon ink injections (as did I), did isolate a serum inhibitory factor and found (as had I) an effect of globulin on the course of infection (see earlier). He also did little biochemistry. That, he left for the post-doctoral. I expected that once I began to work in the lab he would lead me by the hand and demonstrate the use of the culture techniques, but he did not. That would have taken time away from his research. Instead, he provided notes, papers, and oral advice and when needed he asked his technician to assemble the appropriate apparatus. When there were results he would make critical comment, but he never directly interfered in one's research. He regarded us as professional colleagues and when at the outset I called him Dr. Trager he insisted I call him Bill. He taught us to be research scientists by his example.

The Trager laboratory used the bird malaria *P. lophurae*. The infection was maintained by blood passage in ducklings where (unlike that in chickens) the developmental cycles were synchronous, the degree of infection high (as much as 90% of the red cells were infected in four days) and the large body size of the duckling (1–2 kilo) allowed for the possibility of obtaining up to 100 ml of blood from each duckling. Ducklings were kept in rabbit cages fitted with feeding and water troughs in a dark, dank and smelly sub-basement animal room. Duckling droppings are quite watery and so the cages had no paper-lined trays (as was the case with the chickens at Northwestern) instead the feces dropped through the wire flooring of the cage and on to the concrete floor of the animal room. Once a day an animal caretaker dressed in khaki fatigues, rubber boots and a hat made from a brown paper bag went into the duck room and hosed down the entire room, and flushed the feces into a floor drain. Adjoining the duck room was a smaller room used for injecting and drawing blood from the duckling. To withdraw blood from a large duckling required two people. One took the duckling and folded back its wings, placed the animal on a table, stretched out the bird lengthwise, the other plucked the feathers from the neck to expose the large jugular vein and then using a heparin-containing syringe fitted with a needle withdrew the blood. Inoculation of blood into a leg vein required only one person. Trager was allergic to dander from the ducklings and rabbits so that when he had to visit the animal house he placed on his face a stubby filter-containing mask making him look like he had the snout of a pig.

The biochemical equipment in the lab consisted of a brand new Beckman DU spectrophotometer (placed in a broom closet!) which Trager was very anxious be used, an assortment of power supplies for electrophoresis, refrigerated centrifuges, fraction collectors, water baths, incubators, a Klett colorimeter, and so on. When I arrived at Rockefeller he asked, "What are your plans for research?" My research interests were actually quite vague so I replied, "I have no plans." Now he revealed his own plans that were a result of Trager having attended a conference in Florida where the other speakers were Julius Marmur (Brandeis University) and Ernest Bueding (Johns Hopkins University). As early as 1955 Bueding (1910–1986) and his coworkers had shown, using immunologic methods, the "Einheit" in biochemistry did not hold: there was enzyme heterogeneity in blood flukes as well as in the tissues of the host. Of course, in this he was at odds with some of the most influential biochemists of the time. During the meeting Bueding asked Trager: do you think malaria parasites have enzyme heterogeneity?

My first laboratory project at the Institute was to produce malaria parasites free from the confines of the red blood cell. By late July I was preparing gram quantities of pure *P. lophurae* and I was once again extracting malaria pigment and characterizing it spectrophotometrically and immunologically. Trager "volunteered" me to provide Marmur, who was carrying out a survey of the nucleotide base composition of DNA from a variety of protozoans using the "melting" properties of DNA, with a large quantity of erythrocyte-free *P. lophurae*. He also suggested that I do not concern myself with *lophurae* DNA but instead concentrate on the possible heterogeneity of the enzyme lactate dehydrogenase (LDH) in *P. lophurae* and its duckling host.

By 1959 the presence of multiple molecular forms of enzymes (isoenzymes) in various animal and plant tissues had been demonstrated using an overlay method after zone electrophoresis in starch gels and in 1960 Elliot Vesell a post-doctoral fellow in the Rockefeller Institute laboratory of Alexander Bearn was separating LDH isoenzymes electrophoretically by starch gel electrophoresis and then directly visualizing the enzyme in the gel. Not recognizing the barriers that might exist between the various Members laboratories I took the opportunity to visit with Vesell and learned to cook up starch gels, and then, after electrophoresis to stain the LDH isoenzymes. With the help of Vessel and Philip D'Alesandro, who had utilized starch block electrophoresis (and modified from the method of Kunkel and Slater[25]) during his doctoral research, by January 1961 I was able to separate *lophurae* LDH from that of the red blood cell both by starch gel and starch block electrophoresis and to Trager's delight the Beckman DU spectrophotometer was fully utilized.

The *Journal of Experimental Medicine* (*JEM*) is a Rockefeller Institute publication with a reputation for publishing some of the finest work in medical-related subjects including studies in immunology, parasitology, microbiology, and virology. It was the Journal where Avery, McCarty, and McLeod published their landmark paper identifying transforming principle as DNA and set the stage for further work on molecular genetics including the Watson–Crick Model of the DNA double helix. The JEM was the journal in which Trager had published most of his work on malaria. On its Editorial Board was the Nobel laureate Peyton Rous (1879–1970), the distinguished immunologist Henry G. Kunkel (1916–1983) and the pathologist Eugene Opie (1873–1971). As a fellow at the Institute I felt it would be an honor for my work on LDH to be published in the JEM and with Trager's 'blessing' the manuscript (Molecular heterogeneity of lactic dehydrogenase in avian malaria *P. lophurae*) was submitted. It was to be edited by Henry Kunkel. Not hearing of the disposition of the manuscript for several months I contacted Kunkel's editorial office and spoke to his secretary (with whom I had a friendly relationship). In an unusually candid 'behind the scene' conversation she informed me that Kunkel was beside himself and very irritated by the manuscript. I decided to talk directly with Kunkel. I (as a brash kid from the South Bronx) approached him at lunch in the staid Welch Hall where the Members and post docs (wearing their ties and jackets) ate on tables covered with linen tablecloths, and meals were served by waitresses, and said "I am Irwin Sherman and I understand you are unhappy with my manuscript." He looked up from his dessert, spoon held at mouth level, and said "The manuscript is deficient in that it doesn't give enough credit to Elliot Vesell." I rewrote the manuscript and brought the revision to his office. He perused it quickly and once again said it was unsatisfactory again indicating that I had not given Vesell enough credit. I went to Trager and told him of Kunkel's rejection and suggested that he, Kunkel, wanted the manuscript to include a reference to his work on starch block electrophoresis. Trager said, "Irwin, this is certainly not the case, Kunkel could not be so petty." I replied. "Wait and see what happens when I change only one thing in the manuscript, that is, the reference list and add his name." When I brought the revised manuscript to Kunkel's editorial office he quickly leafed through the pages of the manuscript and when he reached the list of references and saw his name said, "This is much better. Now it can be accepted."

Published in the *JEM* in December 1961 it was my first research work of which I was really proud. However, the Kunkel review of my work provided another first for me. It was the first time I ever encountered such pettiness by a distinguished researcher whose ego had to be stroked; the experience, for a time, disillusioned me. But, this would not be the last time for such an experience. Later, there would be other instances where jealousy and competiveness linked with ego would affect the outcome of grant applications and manuscript submission. However, this experience early in my career taught me a valuable lesson: the biases and sensitivity by peers may affect the evaluation of your research. I began to appreciate that scientists are humans with all the frailties of humans; some distinguished or not will have clay feet.

One spring day in 1961, Trager's laboratory had a visit from a young post-doctoral from Brandeis University, Alan Wilson. Wilson, an evolutionary biologist, working in the laboratory of Nathan Kaplan was on his way to the Bronx Zoo to pick up dead birds in the hope of analyzing the LDH in their breast muscles. (He had found that flightless (running) and flying birds have different kinds of LDH). The Kaplan laboratory was actively synthesizing analogs of nicotinamide adenine dinucleotide (NAD) and had found that the ratio of enzymatic activity with NAD and its various analogs (especially the acetyl pyridine NAD) was a very sensitive measure of the differences of various dehydrogenases (especially LDH) in different species and in different organs. Wilson had received some of the frozen *P. lophurae* I had sent to Marmur but found the preparation had lost all its catalytic activity through several freeze-thaw cycles. Hearing of my work with LDH (and knowing that I had supplied Marmur with a sample of 'free' malaria parasites) he invited me to bring a fresh preparation of packed frozen *P. lophurae* to Brandeis and to present a seminar. During that one-day visit to Brandeis it was discovered that *P. lophurae* LDH had an exceptionally high affinity for the acetylpyridine analog of NAD. This proved to be the case for other species of *Plasmodium* and today LDH activity with acetylpyridine-NAD serves as the basis for the diagnostic tests OptiMal and Malstat[26,27] for human malaria infections and also as an immunodiagnostic.[28] It has also been used to measure the adherence of falciparum-infected red cells *in vitro*[29] and sequestration in comatose children.[30]

Another project I pursued at the Rockefeller Institute was an antigenic analysis of the soluble proteins of *P. lophurae* using the newer immunologic methods of immunoelectrophoresis and the double diffusion technique of Ouchterlony. In collaboration with Philip D'Alesandro the quantity and quality of LDH in *Trypanosoma lewisi* was characterized and with Norman Stoll's post-doctoral George Jackson non-specific esterases in the axenically grown nematodes *Neoaplectana glaseri* and *N. carpocapsae* were studied.

Believing that scientific research is a collective activity — of ideas, planning, discovery, luck, and fun — I continued this practice of collaboration for the remainder of my professional life.

iv. Research at the University of California

I was quite happy at the Rockefeller Institute — truly a researcher's paradise. Trager would have liked me to stay on as a post-doctoral for as many years as I desired (and D'Alesandro did), however, I wanted to get out from under his shadow, I wanted my own laboratory, and I wanted an opportunity to teach. I decided I needed to find a setting that would allow me to do both teaching and research: the University.

Not knowing exactly how to find a position in a University I answered a few ads for jobs. One interview I had was at NYU (Uptown), where the Chairman showed me a miserable basement laboratory with abandoned equipment and lamented that he wished he could have shown me a better lab and a salary more than $6,000. I brashly replied, "If the lab were better equipped you probably would have offered me an even lower salary." Needless to say, I did not take the job.

Naively, in the old school manner, I thought the way to obtain a University position was to write to individuals not schools. I wrote to one of my former CCNY professors, Herman T. Spieth, who had taken a position in 1954 as Chairman of the Division of Life Sciences at the then newly established campus of the University of California at Riverside (UCR). By the time I wrote to Spieth he had become the Chancellor at UCR and so he passed my letter on to the Chairman of the Division of Life Sciences, Irwin M. Newell. I was invited to Riverside for an interview. During two days I met with the faculty, and gave a seminar. After the interview at UCR I spent a few days at Northwestern University and then returned to the Rockefeller Institute. Sitting in the office with Trager the phone rang. He answered it and passed the phone to me saying, "It's for you." It was Irwin Newell. Newell asked, "What did you think of UCR?" In a New York attitude I replied, "It was OK." "No," Newell said, "Do you want the job? There are two candidates for the position and I am giving you first choice." I held the palm of my hand over the mouthpiece of the phone and whispered to Trager: "they are offering me the job at Riverside. What shall I do?" He shrugged his shoulders. On impulse, I uncovered the mouthpiece and said, "All right I'll take the job." That was how I joined the UCR faculty.

On June 22, 1962 I was given a farewell party at the Institute and Trager sent me off with a poem: here's to a lad named Irwin/ Who with devotion unswervin/ Cooks up that gel/ Grinds the parasites well/ Finds isoenzymes there by the dirzin.

After I was resident at UCR I discovered some background on the invitation to join the faculty. When Spieth received my letter he passed it on to Newell who asked Spieth what he knew about me. Spieth had kept the grade books from his days at CCNY and told Newell "He took my Field Biology course and did very well." It was on that basis that Newell asked me to interview. Newell made me the job offer, however, there was another candidate for the position, a Canadian electron microscopist, Kenneth Wright, and to this day I am not certain that I was the top choice by the faculty. Indeed, I was never told of the faculty vote and after getting to know Newell better I found on occasion he was inclined to take decisions without full consultation believing he knew best. It was an uncomfortable year when Wright became a post-doctoral in the Division working with the microbiologist Eugene Cota-Robles and I was appointed Assistant Professor at a salary of $7,600. (Two years later Wright left Riverside to become a faculty member at the University of Toronto (Canada), where he remained for his entire career.)

The city of Riverside, California, 60 miles east of Los Angeles (LA), was founded in 1870. It is the birthplace of the citrus industry in the United States. Indeed, the parent navel orange tree still sits at the corner of Arlington and Magnolia Avenues behind a fence. The climate is said to be sub-tropical, but it is more desert-like with very hot summers and a very low (11 inches) annual rainfall. The region is suitable for growing citrus and avocado provided irrigation water is available. In the 1960s much of the acreage of the city was in citrus groves. Riverside is in what was referred to as the 'smog belt' being one of the most polluted areas in all of Southern California. The NY Times referred to it as the site where there is a confluence of two aerial sewers. The city's major employers were March Air Force Base, the University of California, the Country of Riverside, the Riverside Unified School District and the Engineering companies Rohr and Bourns. The downtown area, about 4 miles from campus, has a small museum, a few movie theatres, an art museum, library, department stores, several churches, a world famous hotel, the Mission Inn, and a synagogue. UCR, established in 1954 as a small undergraduate College of Letters and Sciences, is located at the foot of the Box Springs Mountains — really hills that appear like non-descript piles of rubble. Occupying the same site is the Citrus Research Center (CRC) a component of the statewide Agricultural Experiment Station (AES). Although the CRC was established in 1904 at the foot of Mt. Rubidoux it moved to the Box Springs site in 1907. Appropriately, the Air Pollution Research Center is also located on the campus.

En route to Riverside I made a quick visit to the University of Washington where I met one of my heroes of malaria biochemistry, Neal Groman (1920–2011) who confessed to me that after working with bird malaria at the University of Chicago for his Ph. D. (under James Moulder) he never wanted to see another chicken. Luckily, someone left him a virus and that became his life's experimental work. (A common experience of many researchers who worked with bird and monkey malarias in the 1940s and afterwards decided it was just too difficult to maintain the infections, the hosts were noisy, the animal rooms filthy, and there was little funding for malaria research so they left the field as did Groman and Moulder to work on viruses and rickettsiae.)

I arrived in Riverside on a blistering hot day in September 1962. At the time there was commuter air service from LA and when the plane landed at the tiny Riverside airport I was the only passenger leaving the aircraft. My suitcases were deposited on the tarmac and as I walked to the terminal I must have looked (I assume) like Willy Loman in *Death of a Salesman*. It was high noon and as I saw the plane taxi down the runway for takeoff I had a sinking feeling that I had made a grave error in accepting a position at the smallest UC campus (3,000 students) in a small (85,000 population) backwater town on the fringe of the California desert. I took a taxi to the campus and still schlepping my suitcases to the Life Sciences building met, quite by accident, William (Bill) Belser a newly recruited microbiologist from the Scripps Institution of Oceanography in San Diego. He deposited my bags in the Division office and we went to lunch. Thus, began a wonderful 30-year collegial relationship.

I had not arranged for housing in Riverside so I lived for a week at the Mission Inn hotel. This eventually became too expensive so I was given a back bedroom in the home of Carlton Bovell, another microbiologist in the Division, where I slept on a field cot. Eventually I found a one-bedroom apartment not far from campus and purchased a 1962 Corvair Monza. I expected that when I arrived on campus my laboratory would be ready. No such luck. Construction did not begin until after arrival so I spent the next nine months sitting at a desk in the hallway preparing lectures for the two assigned undergraduate courses — Invertebrate

Zoology and Parasitology. When I asked Chairman Newell what he expected me to do in these courses to my surprise he said, "Teach whatever appeals to you and in whatever manner you choose." (Of course, I inherited his 8 a.m. Invertebrate Zoology class and found his laboratory directions to be useless). Initially I was concerned by the lack of guidance, however, it became an opportunity that would allow my creativity to run free. I also had great aspirations for my teaching: I wanted the lectures and laboratory exercises to be engaging experiences that would inspire interest in the subject, not just describe and explain but to provide the students with something of lasting value. I hoped that teaching would be an opportunity for dialogue — a chance for me to learn just as I hoped my students would learn from me. And, I wanted to be critical to the students' fuller comprehension of biology. I expected my lectures to be thought provoking and breezy, not stale or boring. Clearly, I was a naïve optimist.

Based on my positive summer experiences in teaching in the Invertebrate Zoology course at the MBL and the dull aspects of labs in Parasitology at Northwestern University I became convinced the laboratories for both of these courses would engage students only if they were allowed to work with live material. I filled the laboratories in Invertebrate Zoology with exercises using live animals. The Parasitology courses I had taken as a graduate student at Northwestern University consisted almost entirely of pickled specimens or microscopic slides and I felt I (and my classmates) had been deprived of a full appreciation of the dynamic aspects of parasitism. I began asking colleagues in Southern California (principally Gordon Ball and Marietta Voge of UCLA) and elsewhere in the country for some of their research materials — ascarids, trypanosomes, tapeworms, trichomonads, malaria parasites — that could be used in the Parasitology teaching laboratories at UCR. And to my delight they did so.

The students in the Parasitology course I taught were required to carry out independent projects using live parasites in addition to studying the slide collections. The projects were to be written up as if they were to be submitted to a journal for publication. I cannot forget driving with two students to a Farmer Johns packing plant in LA to obtain specimens for one of their projects. Emerging from the plant was a burly man wearing a plastic apron. "What do youse want?" he said. Not wishing to insult him

I said, "*Ascaris lumbricoides* and *Macracantharhynchus hirudinaceous.*" He looked at me perplexed and said, "Do you want da pink ones or da white ones?" We took both as they were squeezed out of a pig's intestines using an old-fashioned washing machine roller. The students did gel electrophoresis of the various worm tissues and found specific protein patterns, some of which might have served as antigens for immunodiagnostic purposes, but regrettably nothing further was done.

One of the first things I had to do to get my research going was to obtain a local source of ducklings. Luckily, Southern California has a large Chinese population that consumes large numbers of white Pekin ducks. Their supplier (and mine) was the Ward Duck Farm in Colton (12 miles from Riverside) and later in La Puente when the Colton Farm with its 25,000 breeder ducks closed down. During my early years at UCR I used *P. lophurae* in ducklings because it allowed us to obtain large quantities of erythrocyte "free" parasites each week very inexpensively. At seminars, in discussing our research, I had a standard line that went: a gram of parasites that costs only a buck a duck. I was convinced (as was Trager) that the *lophurae*-duckling system was an appropriate model for human malaria; moreover it would be another 15 years before *Plasmodium falciparum* would be grown *in vitro* in continuous culture. There was an animal room (with a stainless steel door labelled in bold letters VIVARIUM) on the ground floor of the UCR Life Sciences building that was set aside for my ducks. Initially, housing the larger ducklings was a problem since it would be impossible to reproduce the kind of animal room at the Rockefeller Institute. I designed and the departmental shop built two large bathtubs, partitioned into several compartments each with a mesh wire floor suspended over the bottom of the tub; each cage had a food tray and running the length of the bathtub was a trough of water. The walls of the cage were flushed continuously but to make it really clean and to reduce the smell required a thorough hosing of the tub. In this manner the floor of the animal room remained dry, the ducks had access to water 24 hour a day and under a 12 hour light-12 hour dark cycle the parasites grew synchronously. The tubs lasted 20 years. At first the ducks that died were buried somewhere on campus and later when the Division had an incinerator they were incinerated. Those that survived or had not been infected were taken to Fairmont Park by my technician to be retired or they were used in a duck feast at the Belser's home. To have the ducks dressed I arrived before 8 a.m. in the vivarium and put several live ducks in a gunny sack to be taken to McCall's Poultry. One morning as I was leaving with this quivering sack I met the departmental storekeeper who greeted me but said no more as he looked upon the vibrating sack. I always wondered whether he thought I was disposing of a human body.

My lab-office was on the 2nd floor of the Life Sciences building (later renamed Spieth Hall after UCR's first Chancellor and my former Field Biology instructor at CCNY). It was a room 12' × 30'. No faculty office had its own phone just a buzzer connecting the lab-office to the departmental office on the ground floor. When a phone call came in, I was buzzed, and ran down a flight of stairs to answer the phone in the departmental office.

In 1959, the College of Letters and Sciences at UCR, solely dedicated to undergraduate education, transitioned into a general campus with undergraduate and graduate training and the prospect for professional schools. It was this opportunity to have graduate students that had attracted me to the campus. From 1954–1959 there was a strained relationship between the CRC/AES and the biologists in the Division of Life Sciences. The strain continued during the time I was a new faculty member however I did not find it an impediment and for the most part was able to interact with the CRC biochemists (notably Brian Mudd) and plant scientists (especially Irwin Ting) and to use their equipment and collaborate.

It was expected of University of California faculty that in addition to their teaching assignments that they conduct research and train graduate students. However, since support for laboratory or field research from the University was modest it was essential that one obtain extramural funding in order to mount a vigorous and productive research program. During my first year at UCR I wrote and received a three-year NIH grant to study molecular heterogeneity of enzymes in malaria. There was not much equipment in my UCR lab and the money provided by the department initial complement (amounting to a few thousand dollars) did not go very far. The NIH grant in the amount of ~$20,000 provided monies for my summer salary, a technician's salary, purchase of animals, their feeding as well as funds for reagents. For the summer of 1963 I was appointed as an Instructor in the Invertebrate Zoology course at the MBL with a salary of a few thousand dollars. As a consequence I was able to use the monies allocated by the NIH grant for my summer salary to purchase equipment such as microscopes, incubators, centrifuges, balances, etc. (This was done after approval by the NIH administrator). I continued this practice for the several summers I taught at the MBL. By September 1963, I had hired a laboratory technician, had infected ducklings (sent to me by Trager), a local source of young white Pekin ducklings, and a lab with sufficient equipment to begin to do research. In the first few years at UCR, I could not afford to purchase a spectrophotometer so I had to run downstairs to the microbiology teaching lab where there was a Beckman DU spectrophotometer.

My own involvement with *Plasmodium* DNA began by accident rather than by design. *P. lophurae* had been isolated in 1938 by Lowell T. Coggeshall (of the Rockefeller Foundation) from the blood of a Borneo fireback pheasant, *Lophurae igniti igniti*, kept captive in the Bronx Zoo and thereafter blood was inoculated into chicks and ducks. The growth of *P. lophurae* in young ducklings was phenomenal. Five days after inoculation (by hypodermic syringe) of suitably diluted infected blood almost 90% of the recipients' red blood cells were infected. And, it was possible to obtain 100 ml of whole blood from a single duckling; after spinning in a centrifuge it was possible to obtain 10–20 ml of packed red cells with a wet weight of ~15 gm — an amount equivalent to that from a luxuriant culture of bacteria. At the time purifying an enzyme required fairly large quantities of crude material. *P. lophurae* was perfectly suited for this. By the mid-1960s I had worked out methods for isolating substantial quantities of parasites removed from their hemoglobin-rich habitat — the red blood cell.

As told earlier Trager attended a meeting in Florida where another participant was the Brandeis University molecular biologist Julius Marmur (1926–1996). Marmur following hard on the discovery by the Rockefeller Institute physician Oswald Avery of pneumococcal DNA (called transforming principle) as the genetic material had worked with Avery's colleague, Rollin Hotchkiss (1911–2004), at Rockefeller (above us on the 4th floor of Theobald Smith Hall!) and demonstrated that the

DNA of pneumococcus coded for an enzyme. Later, after developing highly reproducible methods for DNA purification Marmur was able to show that upon heating purified DNA the helical strands separated (called melting) and the melting temperature was dependent on the composition of the DNA, that is, the percent of guanine plus cytosine (G+C). Marmur was attempting to use the melting temperature of DNA from a variety of bacteria to be used "as a valuable asset in their classification." He told Trager he needed some one-celled microbes that were not bacteria for comparative purposes, and he asked whether Trager could help supply these. Trager had no intention of spending his valuable time in preparation of gram quantities of malaria parasites since this would require abandoning his beloved cultures for several days. So he 'volunteered' me to send Marmur some of my samples of *P. lophurae*. I did so and when the results were published I was thanked for 'useful discussions' but unexpectedly the data for the *P. lophurae* DNA was not included. When I asked Marmur about the omission he simply replied, "It was so low in G+C that it didn't fit." Indeed, what Marmur had found was that the malaria parasite G+C content was 20%!

Eight years later, Charles Walsh a graduate student in my UCR laboratory confirmed Marmur's unpublished findings, but our publication received little attention. Others working in malaria biochemistry regarded it to have no real significance since this malaria parasite came from a bird with little in common with the human malaria, *P. falciparum*. It was gratifying many years later, when *P. falciparum* could be grown in culture so its DNA could be analyzed that its % G+C was 18–20% (similar to that of *P. lophurae*) and very different from the malarias infecting rodents and monkeys, which were 24% and 37% respectively.

The research on DNA in my laboratory did more than simply confirm Marmur's work. Walsh was able to show that the nucleus of the duckling red blood cell did not supply precursors for the synthesis of parasite DNA, and although the parasite synthesized pyrimidines *de novo* preformed purines were required. This venture with malaria DNA and nucleic acid metabolism might have led me to join the ranks of the 'gene hunters' however it did not. Rather for the next decade my laboratory continued to study the products of malaria genes — proteins, especially isoenzymes with generous extramural research support from the NIH.

v. Studies of Malaria Antigens

During my time as a post-doctoral fellow at the Rockefeller Institute I read Leslie Stauber's paper[31] on malaria in which he wrote: "some years ago I felt annoyed that I could not do what a canary or a chicken or duckling can do; namely, distinguish between (aside from microscopically) the various species of malaria parasites injected into them." Stauber who was then a Professor of Zoology at Rutgers University was, of course, referring to the malaria parasite antigens and the nature of the host's immune response to these. I too had been concerned with attempts to distinguish clearly host and parasite antigens and had employed the recently developed techniques of protein isolation and characterization to look for relationships between the parasite proteins and the host proteins as well as their role in the development of protective immunity. In my own work I found that although the serum of chickens after immunization with killed parasites produced lines of precipitate (called precipitins) against parasite extracts, no such precipitins were produced in the serum of naturally induced blood infections. I wrote: "precipitins ... bear no relation to immunity ... the titer produced by natural infection without adjuvant is of a transitory nature and of low titer so that no precipitation occurs. Vaccination by the use of killed parasites plus adjuvant does not seem a practical means, as yet, for protection against malaria."[32] My studies on malaria antigens were contemporaneous with those of a group headed by Avivah Zuckerman, in Israel.

Avivah Zuckerman (1915–1977) was born in New York City. The Zuckermans, fierce Zionists, emigrated to Palestine in 1925. However, when Avivah took ill they were forced to return to New York where she could be properly treated and in 1932 she received a B.S. from Hunter College. The Zuckerman returned to Palestine where Avivah enrolled in the Hebrew University becoming one of the first students in bacteriology (M.S. 1938). In 1940 she was enrolled as a doctorate student under W. H. Taliaferro (1895–1973) at the University of Chicago. Taliaferro, trained as a classical physiologist studying the eye of planaria, had a genius for turning unafraid to a new field and bringing to bear upon it unusual insight. When Avivah became his student he was concerned with cellular and humoral (antibody) factors in host–parasite relationships. He and his students concentrated on laboratory infections that could be controlled and experimentally attacked. Avivah studied infections in the bird malaria *P. gallinaceum* and developed immunologic tests (including precipitins) to measure immunity. She received the Ph.D. in 1944, spent a few years as an Instructor in Bacteriology and Parasitology at the University of Chicago, and after 1946 was on the faculty of the Hebrew University in Jerusalem. In 1960, Avivah observed: in human malaria the total loss of blood is more extensive than can be attributed to the direct rupture of red blood cells by parasites. She suggested that the surface of the infected red blood cell may be altered by the parasites to become antigenic and that this may then result in the production of autoantibody and removal of the antibody-coated red cells by the spleen caused the anemia. It would be decades later that my laboratory would discover the membrane changes in the infected red cells that would alter those red blood cells antigenically (see Chapter 9), however, in contrast to her speculation we concluded these changes would not result in anemia but instead in protection.

Because malaria had exacted a heavy toll on U.S. troops during both World Wars as well as the Korean conflict the Department of Defense, and in particular The Naval Medical Research Institute (NMRI) and the Walter Reed Army Institute of Research (WRAIR), established and maintained active malaria research programs dedicated for protecting the health of U.S. military personnel. In 1963 Elvio Sadun (1918–1974), Chief of Medical Zoology and Special Assistant to the Director for Basic Research at WRAIR, recognized the need for basic research on malaria and he helped to establish a program to develop new prophylactic and therapeutic drugs for malaria. He organized an *International Panel Workshop on the Cultivation of Plasmodium and the Immunology of Malaria* (August 27–29, 1963). The stated objective was to summarize the available information, explore new approaches and delineate problems. The most pressing need was to attract researchers to work on malaria. I was invited to participate in the Workshop where I was invited to comment on the work of Avivah Zuckerman and at the conclusion of the meeting she invited me to visit Israel.

In 1964, I was attending the meeting of the Society of Protozoologists in Rome, and decided afterwards to go Israel and visit with Avivah. However, before that I wanted to see the pyramids and Sphinx in Cairo,

Egypt. Getting into Israel from Egypt was an adventure. (And I loved adventure). At the time, before the six-day 1967 Arab–Israeli War, Jerusalem was in Jordan. Before my departure for Rome my Riverside travel agent had not informed me that in order to enter Israel from Egypt I had to spend three calendar days in Jordan. (I had planned to be in transit in Amman, Jordan and then enter Israel via Jerusalem). The Arab states did not recognize the State of Israel so there was no way to contact Avivah of my delay. I arranged for a hotel in Jordan, and took the time while in Jordan to visit the Old City of Jerusalem, walked the Stations of the Cross, the Garden at Gethsemane and visited Bethlehem. On the third day in Jordan I applied to leave; this was granted and carrying my suitcase I crossed the border from Jordan into Israel via the Mandelbaum Gate. When I did arrive a few days later than expected, and Avivah expressed concern about what had happened, we had long conversations about the conditions in the Old City of Jerusalem. I didn't realize that she had served as an officer in the Israeli Defense Army (Hagana), that she and her family were friends to the Israeli Prime Ministers Golda Meier and David Ben Gurion and she was a poet. She also told me stories of how difficult life was in Israel before Independence and her unflinching pride in all that had been accomplished. We talked science until the wee hours of the morning focusing on protective antigens and the causes of malaria anemia (autoimmunity).

Shortly before her untimely death in 1977 of breast cancer Zuckerman and her collaborators had published more than 100 papers on malaria immunity, autoimmunity, and malaria antigens. Her broad knowledge of malaria immunity was demonstrated in 1969, with a five-year review of the *Current Status of the Immunology of Malaria and of the Antigenic Analysis of Plasmodia*,[33] and again in a posthumously published review of the literature entitled, *Current status of the immunology of blood and tissue protozoa II. Plasmodium.*[34] These publications were exceedingly valuable contributions for those of us who would work on vaccines.

The day-to-day business of science consists not in hunting for facts but in testing hypotheses. In 1973 when I studied the nature of the malaria parasite ribosome I was testing a hypothesis (although it was paraded as a fact by Joseph and Judith Ilan). I first met Joseph Ilan when I attended a meeting on *Experimental Malaria* at WRAIR in May 1969. Joseph announced to the assembled group of biochemists and immunologists that he had solved the raison d' etre for *Plasmodium* being a parasite i.e. it stole a part of the host red blood cell ribosome.[35] It made absolutely no sense to me since during parasite feeding the red cell ribosomes would surely have been digested entirely; further, most mature red blood cells — where malaria parasites live and grow — lack ribosomes.

I applied for and received a fellowship from the NIH for a 1973–1974 sabbatical leave. The project was to test the validity of the Ilans work (i.e. a hypothesis masquerading as fact) on the biogenesis of the malaria ribosome. I applied to work at the National Institute for Medical Research (NIMR) in London (Mill Hill) and was accepted. James (Jim) Williamson (1918–1993) arranged housing in Mill Hill just downhill from the NIMR. I met Jim 10 years earlier when out of the blue, I was invited by Anthony Allison (who first described the protective effects of sickle cell trait on malaria) to present a paper on glucose-6-phosphate dehydrogenase in malaria at the Seventh International Congress on Tropical Medicine and Malaria in Rio de Janeiro, Brazil (September 1–11, 1963) and there I met Jim. From 1954–1960 Jim, whose primary interest was in chemotherapy worked at the West African Institute for Trypanosomiasis Research in Nigeria and in 1960 joined the NIMR in London where he remained until his death working on malaria and trypanosome biochemistry. Jim was a balding Scot with a bushy moustache; wire rimmed glasses and thick Scottish accent. He was an original and productive researcher, always full of ideas, had a critical knowledge of the literature and a scant regard for most current received opinion, a disregard for the artificial boundaries for scientific thought and action and an irreverent sense of humor. When the Nobel Laureate Peter Medawar (and his chief at NIMR) wrote his opus magnum, *The Art of the Soluble*, Jim quipped: "ah ha but soluble in what?" His conversation was laced with good natured and humorous observation, and he loved to party. We had a wonderful evening together in Rio. Jim introduced me to all the right people at NIMR, as well as single malt scotch and almost every day we had a pub lunch together and talked research.

At the NIMR I rubbed shoulders with the other members of the Parasitology Section: Peter Trigg, Peter Shakespeare, Iain Wilson, and Neil Brown. After a few days of not doing anything I prevailed upon Peter Trigg to introduce me to the local ribosome expert R. A. (Bob) Cox and his able technician Betty Higginson. As a guest at the NIMR I was without a technician or administrative responsibilities and so could focus all my attention on doing experiments. Betty taught me to isolate ribosomes from rabbit reticulocytes (which was Cox's experimental material) and then thanks to Peter Trigg I was able to obtain *P. knowlesi* from infected rhesus monkeys (which were available at the NIMR and which Peter wrestled to the ground and anesthetized so blood could be drawn). On my own I developed methods for isolating the *knowlesi* ribosomes (which took all day) and at day's end all I had at the bottom of a centrifuge tube was a dirty brown smudge. When I proudly showed this to Cox (who did no lab work himself) he sneered saying, "If that's all you can get I'd go back to rabbits." (With the anemic rabbits produced by injections of phenylhydrazine it was possible to get grams of ribosomes but these would do me no good since they would be different from malaria parasite ribosomes and I was interested in malaria not rabbits). I found the ribosomes of *knowlesi* to be different from those of the rabbit reticulocyte, to be intact and not derived from the host red cell.[36] The Ilans "hypothesis" was incorrect. Years later the Ilans corrected the mistake ascribing their erroneous findings to ribosome degradation by an enzyme. At NIMR I was able to use the *knowlesi* ribosomes to develop a cell-free protein synthesizing system that allowed for the *in vitro* testing of antimalarials on protein synthesis.[37] Later, in the laboratory at UCR we would use these ribosomes for their potential as a vaccine (see p. 75).

Returning to UCR, I with my technician, Lynn Jones, adapted the method I had used for *P. knowlesi* ribosome isolation to *P. lophurae*.[38] Despite my now being Chairman of the Department of Biology the NIH-supported research in the laboratory continued at an accelerated pace and by the late 1970s my reputation as a malaria biochemist had been solidified. In 1979 I published a seminal paper entitled, *The Biochemistry of Plasmodium*.[39] I was invited to become a member of the WHO Steering Committee for the Chemotherapy of Malaria where I continued to hone my critical skills by reviewing hundreds of grant applications. In my own laboratory I applied the tools and concepts learned in other fields to investigations of malaria. I held myself to a very high standard and felt that I would not publish any work that was not consonant with the best of my intellect, and with emphasis on accuracy, reproducibility, and a critical interpretation of the data. I put a premium on accomplishment and originality. These were the values I instilled in the graduate students and post-doctoral fellows who spent time in my laboratory and my hope was that they would practice this after leaving.

In the 1960s there was relatively little competition in malaria research from other laboratories, however, by the 1970s with increased funding from the U.S. Army, WHO, USAID, and NIH more and more biochemists began to enter the malaria field. Unfortunately most of these biochemists/cell biologists lacked an appreciation for the idiosyncrasies of malaria parasites and this served to confuse rather than enhance our understanding of the biochemistry of *Plasmodium*. And, in the late 1970s when the rage amongst biochemists was membranes, membranes, membranes I began to think my laboratory should also focus on the molecular characteristics of the parasite and red cell membranes. We asked two simple questions: how did the membranes differ from one another and of what importance are such differences to parasitism? Initially, we were not thinking of vaccines, but it wouldn't be long before we too embarked on a quest for a malaria vaccine and in this we were in competition with other investigators.

Chapter 3
Taming the Malaria Parasite

It is difficult to minimize the contributions of vaccines to human health. There are vaccines against disease-causing viruses and bacteria. Some of these vaccines contain inactivated viruses (yellow fever, rabies, polio, measles, rubella, chicken pox, shingles) and some are made from killed microbes (hepatitis A, typhoid, cholera, plague, pertussis, Japanese encephalitis), and there are vaccines consisting of purified proteins or polysaccharides (hepatitis B, human paillomavirus, diphtheria, pertussis, tetanus (DPT), anthrax, *Streptococcus pneumoniae, Hemophilus influenzae, Neisseria meninigitis*) derived from pathogenic microbes. Not one of these vaccines could have been made without a laboratory source of the microbe — growing in chick embryos, others growing in tissue culture cells and some multiplying in cell-free cultures. Likewise, the preparation of a malaria vaccine would require a laboratory source of parasites.

From 1947 onwards Trager at the Rockefeller Institute maintained *P. lophurae*-infected red cells obtained from infected ducklings using the Harvard rocker dilution method. The culture system consisted of red blood cells suspended in the nutrient "Harvard" medium, gently rocked to simulate blood flow, and gassed with humidified 5% CO_2 + 95% air. Under these conditions continuous culture was not obtained. Periodically, he tried the same system with *Plasmodium falciparum*-infected red cells. Under these conditions parasite growth was less than optimal and reinvasion rates by merozoites were low so that continuous culture of the parasites could not be achieved. In 1971 Trager decided to abandon the

63

rocker-dilution method and to substitute a perfusion system in which the culture medium would flow gently over a settled layer of cells. His reasoning was this: since *P. falciparum*-infected red cells spend most of their 48 hour developmental cycle attached to the walls of the post-capillary venules (i.e. sequestration), agitation of the infected red cells might be detrimental to parasite growth and invasion. As a result, blood was removed from a night owl (*Aotus*) monkey infected with the Falciparum Oak Knoll (FVO) strain of *P. falciparum* (obtained from Trager's former postdoctoral Wasim Siddiqui who at the time was working at Stanford University), the red blood cells were washed, diluted with human AB red blood cells suspended in 15% human serum and placed in "flow vials," and a variety of tissue culture media were screened. The newly developed RPMI 1640 medium was found to be superior to all others tested. Trager also changed the gas mixture from 5% CO2 + 95% air to 7% CO_2 + 5% O_2 + 88% N_2. Under these conditions, and with a settled layer of red cells from a 2–8% red blood cell suspension, it was possible to keep the parasites growing and reproducing for 24 days by adding fresh uninfected red blood cells every 3–4 days.[50]

In 1966 the United States Agency for International Development (USAID) funded a project for the development of a malaria vaccine at the University of Illinois (under Paul Silverman) and by the mid-1970s when USAID decided to diversify and expand its vaccine effort it enlisted the support of Trager to undertake the cultivation of *P. falciparum*. In his proposal to USAID Trager specifically asked for funds to support a post-doctoral who was experienced in the cultivation of intracellular parasites. James B. Jensen (b. 1943) was invited by Trager to fill that position.

In January 1976, and shortly after Jensen's arrival at the Rockefeller Institute (now named Rockefeller University) Trager and he planned their approach to cultivating *P. falciparum*: first, they selected commercially available culture media high in glucose, second, they abandoned the Harvard medium bicarbonate buffer system (since it was clearly inadequate to control the lactic acidosis), third they decided to compare parasite growth in the rocker flasks and "flow vials," and fourth, they elected to modify the gas mixture. During February 1976, they tested the suitability of commercial media using falciparum-infected red blood cells from an *Aotus* monkey. The parasites in the rocker flask died out within four days, but after the same period of time the parasite numbers were maintained in the flow vial. The numbers of parasites increased dramatically in the flow vials when fresh red cells were added to a diluted sample of infected red blood cells, but attempts to maintain parasites in the rocker flasks failed time and time again. In the meantime Jensen decided to take some of the infected red cells and place them into 35 mm Petri dishes with a variety of media (such as RPMI 1640 and Dulbecco's Modified Eagles Medium, Ham's H-12, MEM and Medium 199). When he placed the Petri dishes containing the infected red cells into a 5% CO_2/air incubator the parasites died out after 2–3 days. It was then that Jensen decided to employ a candle jar instead of the CO_2 incubator — a method he had previously used to grow cells for the cultivation of various coccidian species (and when the CO_2 cell culture incubators in the virology lab at Utah State were unavailable to him). Jensen located a large glass desiccator, placed his Petri dish cultures inside, and after lighting a candle, closed the stopcock; this was incubated at 37°C for several days.[40] At first Trager was dismayed to observe Jensen's use of a 19th century technology, but when he was shown the Giemsa-stained slides Trager was convinced Jensen was on to something. In the summer of 1976 Milton Friedman, a graduate student in the Trager lab who was working in the MRC laboratories in The Gambia, arranged for a sample of human blood infected with *P. falciparum* to be sent to New York. This was diluted with RPMI 1640 (which turned out to be the best of the commercial media) in Petri dishes, placed in a candle jar and incubated. The line grew very well and became FCR-3 (Falciparum Culture Rockefeller), one of the most widely used strains.[52]

The successful continuous cultivation of *P. falciparum* involved more than an understanding of the idiosyncratic growth requirements of *Plasmodium* it needed determination and the combined talents of two exceptional culturists. Jensen, however, remained largely in the shadows and most of the glory was showered on Trager, who received many honors including the Manson Medal of the Royal Society of Tropical Medicine and Hygiene, the Leuckart Medal, the S.T. Darling Medal of the World Health Organization, the Augustine Le Prince Medal of the American Society for Tropical Medicine and Hygiene and Thailand's Prince Mahidol Award; he was elected to the prestigious National Academy of Sciences (USA) and received honorary degrees from Rockefeller University and Rutgers University.

The continuous culture of *P. falciparum* dramatically altered studies of malaria parasites. It could be usefully applied in nearly every aspect of research: chemotherapy, drug resistance, pathogenesis, gametocytogenesis, mosquito transmission, genetics, and provided the necessary material for the development of vaccines. Perhaps most importantly the continuous laboratory culture of *P. falciparum* made possible molecular approaches including the sequencing the entire genome that enabled a giant leap forward in understanding the biochemical properties of *Plasmodium* and allowed for identification and production of putative vaccine candidates.

Chapter 4

The Quest for a Blood Stage Vaccine Begins

The concept of a blood stage vaccine for *Plasmodium falciparum* is based on a fundamental principle: mimic the immunity that occurs in nature. In malaria-endemic areas natural acquired immunity is induced by continued exposure to the bite of falciparum-infected anopheline mosquitoes and although blood parasites persist, successive bouts of clinical disease are diminished due to reduced parasite multiplication and growth. The assumption of proponents of a blood stage vaccine against falciparum malaria is that it will accelerate the acquisition of acquired immunity, inhibit parasite invasion into red blood cells and affect parasite multiplication to reduce the parasite burden thereby limiting disease severity and death. Such a vaccine would offer an enormous benefit to the public health, particularly infants and children living in malaria endemic areas who suffer the most.

The quest for a blood stage vaccine for malaria began in the early 1940s when Henry R. Jacobs a Northwestern University physician showed that ducklings vaccinated with insoluble extracts of *P. lophurae* when mixed with a staphylococcus toxoid (that had been used to make non-antigenic materials more antigenic) resulted in increased protection of four out of six ducklings against challenge.[41] He concluded the need for the toxoid was that the parasite material on its own did not efficiently provoke antibody production. Jacobs' work suggested to Jules Freund

(1890–1960), whose name today is remembered for his adjuvant (from the Latin word *adjuvare* meaning "to aid") techniques for immunization that a blood stage vaccine might be possible if the potency of the malarial antigens could be enhanced.

Jules Freund, born in Budapest, Hungary, received his MD at the Royal Hungarian University, served in the Austrian Army (1913–1914), held several public health positions and then immigrated to the United States in 1923 to work at the Antitoxin and Vaccine Laboratory of Harvard University. He then joined the group of Eugene Opie (the former Johns Hopkins medical student, who along with William MacCallum, recognized the significance of Laveran's flagellum) in the Department of Pathology at the Cornell Medical School in New York. In 1943 Freund became Chief of the Division of Applied Immunology at the newly established Public Health Research Institute of the City of New York. Robert Koch was long dead when Freund began to work on developing an adjuvant, but it was Koch's work on a tuberculosis vaccine that provided an essential ingredient to the successful demonstration that a malaria vaccine was possible.

For his discoveries of the germs of tuberculosis (1882) and that of cholera (1883) the Imperial Government of Germany rewarded Koch by appointment (1885) as Professor of Hygiene in the newly established Hygiene Institute of the University of Berlin. For several years after his appointment, Koch ceased to do research with his own hands and instead relied on his laboratory assistants to do the bench work. Then sometime in 1889 there was an abrupt change in behavior. He was back in the laboratory, doing work with his own hands behind closed doors and speaking to no one for days. In 1890, at the Tenth International Congress of Medicine held in Berlin, Koch made a world-shattering announcement of a "remedy" for tuberculosis. The stolid and cool Koch approached the podium, peered over his gold-rimmed glasses, shuffled his papers, and addressed the crowd: "my discovery of the tubercle bacillus led me to seek substances that would be therapeutically useful against tuberculosis. In spite of many failures I continued my quest and ultimately found a substance, which I call tuberculin, which halted the growth of the tubercle bacteria not only in test tubes but also in animal bodies. Guinea pigs, highly susceptible to tuberculosis, even if they already have the disease in

an advanced state, when injected with tuberculin have the disease halted."
He concluded the lecture: "tuberculin is a cure for tuberculosis!" What
Koch had found was that a glycerin extract of a pure culture of tubercle
bacteria when injected under the skin of a guinea pig resulted in a remark-
able immunologic response. After a delay of one or two days the guinea
pig showed a local or systemic reaction whose severity was dependent on
the amount of tuberculin injected and the host's immunity. The site near
the injection became red, swollen, tender, and ulcerated; it oozed pus
and the lymph nodes enlarged. Despite the fact that at the time of his
announcement of tuberculin therapy Koch had tested it only in guinea
pigs, public and political pressure encouraged testing in human subjects.
These tests soon showed that the therapy was not only useless it was on
occasion fatal. The failure of tuberculin therapy to cure tuberculosis led
Koch to become grumpy, quiet, and restless. He offered his microbe hunting services to countries around the world in the hope of conquering
plagues. During sojourns in Italy and Africa he hunted the malaria parasite
and the means by which it was transmitted and in these endeavors he
failed. Ironically, however, his failed "remedy" — tuberculin — in the
hands of Freund would find success in trials of a protective malaria
vaccine.

As early as 1913 Freund had developed a special interest in hypersen-
sitivity in guinea pigs injected with the substance tuberculin. He found
that guinea pigs sensitized with tubercle bacilli in paraffin oil produced
large quantities of antibodies to the bacteria. This discovery led to the idea
that the oil might act as an adjuvant. Freund and coworkers incorporated
formaldehyde-killed *P. lophurae* combined with a lanolin-like substance,
paraffin oil, and killed tubercle bacteria to vaccinate two-month-old white
Pekin ducklings. (Older ducks weighing 2–3 kilograms were used because
the experiment required a period of at least two months from the time of
first vaccination to challenge, and since these were probably age-immune
the challenge dose had to be high, i.e. 1–5 billion parasitized red blood
cells to produce a lethal infection in control birds). After three injections
given four weeks apart and challenged with blood stage parasites by intravenous inoculation one month after the last immunizing injection seven
out of eight vaccinated ducks survived in contrast to 50% mortality in the
control birds. The survivors, however, had a few parasites in the blood.[42]

In a more extensive study Freund and coworkers found that when vaccinated ducks received two injections of vaccine none died of malaria; they also found, however, that four out of five developed a low-grade blood infection. With a single vaccination there was also evidence of protection, and this seemed to persist for several months. Although protection could be achieved without adjuvant, it was of relatively short duration. This demonstrated that it was possible to produce immunity to malaria without a prior infection, however, immunization did not prevent the duckling from becoming infected altogether. In addition, inoculations had to be done intramuscularly, and protection appeared to be related to adjuvant-induced local tissue reactions, i.e. suppurating pus-filled sores that at times were severe. Freund's experiments clearly demonstrated that vaccination against malaria could be achieved (but only when a suitable and potent adjuvant was used).

In 1932, Sinton and Mulligan isolated a malaria parasite from a long-tailed Malayan kra monkey (*Macaca irus* = *M. fascicularis*) imported from Singapore to Calcutta. It was maintained at the Malaria Institute of India (Delhi) in rhesus monkeys and named *P. knowlesi*, after the Director of the Institute Robert Knowles. In 1932 Knowles and Das Gupta succeeded in experimentally transmitting *P. knowlesi* from monkey to human and then from human to human by inoculation of infected blood. In the early 1930s (and before the advent of penicillin) this monkey malaria was widely used for the treatment of general paralysis of the insane, tertiary syphilis being one of the main reasons for admission to neuropsychiatric institutions. But it soon became apparent that this infection could become uncontrollable and after several fatalities its use was discontinued in favor of the less virulent *P. vivax*.

In 1939, Monroe D. Eaton and Lowell T. Coggeshall working in the Rockefeller Foundation Laboratories in New York City found that immunization of rhesus monkeys with *P. knowlesi* killed by heat, freezing, and thawing or formalin or drying produced no resistance to challenge by live parasites. By contrast, repeated reinfection of chronically infected monkeys enhanced the potency of immune serum and when this serum was injected into animals with an acute infection it had a variable but generally depressing effect on the course of infection if administered in daily doses; relatively large amounts of immune serum given shortly before or at the time of injection of parasites, however, had only a minor effect. The protective effect of immune serum was more marked when the challenge was with 10 *P. knowlesi* parasites than with 1,000 parasites, and protection was more effective when immune serum was incubated with the parasites before injection and given daily during the incubation period and the first stages of infection; if administered after parasites appeared in the blood, however, it was more difficult to protect the monkey with immune serum. Thus, survival or death of the Rhesus monkey was dependent both on the amount of immune serum and the number of *P. knowlesi* parasites used for challenge.[43]

The serum protection experiments of Eaton and Coggeshall were based on work that had been done in in the late-1800s. In 1883 Edwin Klebs and Friedrich Loeffler working in the laboratory of Robert Koch in Berlin, Germany isolated the microbe causing the deadly disease diphtheria when they took swabs from the throat of an infected child. They were able to grow the bacterium in pure culture and named it *Corynebacterium diphtheriae*. Five years later Emile Roux and Alexandre Yersin of the Pasteur Institute in Paris found that the broth in which the *Corynebacterium* were growing contained a substance that produced all the symptoms of diphtheria when injected into a rabbit; at a high enough dose it killed the rabbit. The killing agent was a poisonous toxin. In 1906 Jules Bordet and Octave Gengou identified the specific bacterium causing whooping cough, named it *Bordatella pertussis*, and found that in culture these bacteria produced another kind of toxin, one different from the diphtheria toxin. In 1885 Arthur Nocolaier discovered the tetanus bacillus *Clostridium tetanae* and in 1889 Shibasaburo Kitasato working in Koch's laboratory grew it in pure culture and found the culture fluid contained another kind of toxin. Then in 1890 Emil von Behring and Kitasato, both working with Robert Koch in Berlin found that if small amounts of the tetanus toxin were injected into rabbits the rabbit serum contained a substance that would protect another animal from a subsequent lethal dose of toxin. They called the toxin-neutralizing substance "immune serum." Von Behring found the same thing with the diphtheria toxin. In effect, by toxin inoculation the rabbit had been protected against disease. This process was called vaccination to honor the work of the English physician Edward Jenner who discovered the means for protecting against smallpox using the cowpox virus (*Vaccinia*). The immune protection seen by von Behring and Kitasato could be transferred to another animal by injection of immune serum. In other words it was possible to have 'passive immunity' that is immunity could be borrowed from an animal that had been immunized with the active foreign substance when the serum was transferred by injection to a non-immunized animal. The implications of the research on immune serums for treating human disease were quite obvious to von Behring and others in the Berlin laboratory. Without waiting for the identification and isolation of the active ingredient in immune serum the German government began to support the construction of factories to produce different kinds of immune sera against a wide range of bacterial toxins. Clinical trials were organized first in Germany, then in the rest of Europe and the United States. Initially it was believed that all bacterial infections could be treated by antitoxin immune therapy, but unfortunately only the bacteria that cause diphtheria, pertussis, and tetanus and a few others that produce toxins can be treated this way so the therapeutic application of immune serum against most bacterial infections remains limited.

Paul Ehrlich (1854–1914) working in Koch's lab found that although the diphtheria toxin lost its poisoning capacity with storage it still retained its ability to induce immune serum. He called this altered toxin (nowadays produced by treating with formalin) 'toxoid.' Even today, toxoids made from diphtheria, pertussis, and tetanus toxins are used as the childhood vaccine DPT and is the standard means for eliminating the scourge of these diseases in many countries.

Armed with Emil von Behring's demonstration that immunity stemmed from antibodies to toxins in the serum, and the protection afforded by passive transfer of immune serum by Eaton and Coggeshall, Michael Heidelberger (1888–1991) was optimistic that a malaria vaccine could be developed for humans. As Professor of Immunochemistry at Columbia University and under a contract recommended by the Committee on Medical Research funded by the Office of Scientific Research between 1942–1945, he and a graduate student, Manfred Mayer, prepared a vaccine from *P. vivax*-infected red blood cells obtained from malaria-infected troops who had returned to the United States from the South Pacific and volunteered to donate blood. They used *P. vivax* because it was "safe" — it usually did not cause serious or fatal infections and it had been used for decades in the treatment of those with late-stage syphilis. Blood containing large, hemozoin-laden parasites were used as the starting material; this was treated with dilute formaldehyde, lysed by freezing and thawing and "purified" by centrifugation. To process a pint of blood took 15–20 hours! Using this material Heidelberger conducted the first controlled active immunization studies for vivax malaria. Some 200 volunteer patients suffering from chronic relapsing vivax malaria were divided into three groups. One group received routine therapy, a second group received normal red blood cell membranes, and the third group received the vaccine, consisting of 2–4 billion formaldehyde-killed parasites administered by intracutaneous, subcutaneous, and intravenous routes in divided doses over a period of 4–5 consecutive days. The relapse rate in the three groups was the same. They also administered formaldehyde-killed sporozoites to healthy volunteer inmates, and again this vaccine had no effect on susceptibility to infection by the bite of vivax-infected mosquitoes. Heidelberger concluded the experiments to be "a complete failure" and he never again worked on a vaccine for malaria.[44]

Heidelberger's disappointing findings for a malaria vaccine were in direct contrast to those of Freund and coworkers, who extended their work with bird malaria to *P. knowlesi* in the rhesus monkey.[45] In a preliminary trial each dose was divided into three or five equal portions, injected into the subcutaneous tissues of the neck, armpits, groin, and neck, and then the monkeys were challenged with infected blood. In one of seven vaccinated monkeys no parasites were seen in blood smears and in the others there were fewer than 10 parasites per 100 red blood cells; in the latter case the numbers declined until none could be seen. There were palpable masses at the injection site although these did not ulcerate. In a more extensive study[46] the vaccinated animals developed low grade infections, and none died from malaria when challenged; the low grade blood infection was of short duration and there were no relapses for as long as six months. It was not possible to substitute for the killed tubercle bacteria, however, and when peanut oil was used instead no protection occurred. When killed parasites in saline were injected or when tubercle bacteria were replaced by alcohol–ether extracts of the bacilli or cholesterol or lecithin there was no protection. The titer of complement fixing antibodies was higher in monkeys vaccinated with adjuvant than in those without adjuvant; there was no exact correlation, however, between immunity and the titers of sera. Of the three monkeys vaccinated two died of malaria and the course of the disease was similar to controls and the third monkey developed a low-grade infection lasting 28 days and death occurred on day 34.

Freund's ability to protect ducks and monkeys against challenge by blood stage malaria parasites and the demonstrated need for an adjuvant to immunize against such infections did not have an immediate impact on the development of malaria vaccines. Indeed, it was 20 years later that Targett and Fulton[47] confirmed Freund's findings using formaldehyde-fixed erythrocyte free *P. knowlesi* and infected red cells emulsified in Freund's complete antigen (FCA), the latter being more immunogenic. Vaccination was carried out with an interval of 6–8 weeks between injections with or without adjuvant and the monkeys challenged six weeks after the second vaccination. Of the seven animals vaccinated either with parasites or infected red cells with FCA, no blood stage parasites were seen in three of the monkeys, whereas three others showed a low grade infection that persisted for 23 days after challenge; the remaining animal had a more severe infection but recovered. Four weeks later none of the vaccinated monkeys showed parasites in the blood. Without FCA there was no protection; intramuscular inoculation was found to be more effective in protection than subcutaneous. Although there was a marked increase in serum γ-globulin, this increase was not correlated with protection. Further, an increase in the antibody titer did not correlate with functional immunity in every case suggesting that much of the γ-globulin increase was non-specific[48] something I (and others) had found earlier with the bird malarias (see p. 37).

Partially successful production of non-living vaccines titillates the imagination, and although successful vaccination of birds and monkeys with whole parasites had been achieved (i.e. Freund's work) there had been no identification of a protective antigen. Then, in 1974, as Araxie Kilejian was working with *P. lophurae* in Trager's Rockefeller University laboratory (and before he and Jensen were able to continuously culture *P. falciparum*) she serendipitously discovered a possible protective antigen. Kilejian was trying to isolate nuclei from *P. lophurae*. The parasites were broken open by sound waves and the crude suspension was separated into several fractions by sedimentation in a centrifuge. When each of the fractions was examined with a transmission electron microscope the nuclear fraction showed a great enrichment of electron dense granules. When the isolated granules were dissolved in acetic acid and analyzed they were found to contain a protein with an unusually high amount (~70%) of the amino acid histidine. It was called the histidine-rich protein, or HRP.[49]

Although the dense granules (as well as malaria pigment) are discarded when the *P. lophurae*-infected red cells burst and merozoites are released Kilejian could not countenance that the parasite would expend energy synthesizing a waste product. Using radioactive histidine she found trophozoites and merozoites to accumulate radioactivity and this led her to hypothesize that the HRP was a component of "the polar organelles of merozoites and function in their penetration of erythrocytes." The next "logical" experiment she carried out was to vaccinate ducklings with HRP. Kilejian observed that three out of four ducks showed low-grade infections, indicating a "protective immune response without the use of adjuvant." Two weeks after challenge one of the ducks was used to obtain a globulin preparation, and this was used to transfer protection passively. All ducklings survived, and when these were challenged two and four weeks later they showed "total resistance."[50] Here is where I came on the scene. It made no sense to me that the HRP would serve as a protective vaccine since massive amounts of HRP would be released into the circulation with each parasite reproductive cycle. If anything by such exposure ducklings should be immune i.e. self-cure but in my experience they were not. For several years I too had tried to identify protective antigens in *P. lophurae*, and in this pursuit the immunologist Vincent McDonald joined me. Vincent was making some progress with a parasite ribosomal protein preparation when I suggested that he compare his "protective" antigens to the HRP. Together we carried out an extensive study on HRP trying as best we could to repeat Kilejian's work precisely, but failed.[51] We published our negative findings in the journal *Experimental Parasitology*[52] and Kilejian (clearly irate) submitted a letter stating that we had not in fact repeated her work.[53] We responded with a rebuttal claiming that Kilejian's success could be traced to her using age-immune ducks, too few experimental animals for statistical analysis, and categorically stated HRP played no role in protection. We suggested she repeat the experiments[52]; neither she, however, nor any other laboratory did. I do not know whether my refusal to suppress publication of our research results led to Kilejian leaving the field of malaria research, however, that is just what happened.

The conclusions to be drawn from the immunization studies using bird and monkey malarias are inescapable: protection could be achieved after vaccination with the various stages of the parasite, although, in most instances this required the use of an adjuvant. More often than not the protection achieved was non-sterilizing i.e. there were some parasites in the blood. And, finally in spite of the promise of vaccination a protective malaria antigen had not been identified.

Chapter 5

Malaria Vaccines and Malfeasance

In 1955, full of hubris, the 8th World Health Organization (WHO) Assembly meeting in Geneva, Switzerland, endorsed a policy of global eradication of malaria with reliance on chloroquine treatment and DDT spraying. No mention was made about conducting research that might lead to a protective vaccine. Indeed, there were serious reservations for a malaria vaccine for humans based on clinical, logistical, and economic considerations. Because (as had been noted by Robert Koch more than a century ago) immunity to malaria in humans develops slowly and incompletely, the assumption was that vaccination would not improve on the immunity developed by repeated severe infections. There was also the belief that problems would arise with the acceptability of a vaccine for children within a target population. And finally, some contended that a malaria vaccine would not only be costly to develop, it could serve only as an adjunct to the inexpensive and effective insecticides and antimalarial drugs.

However, by the 1960s, many parts of the world where eradication had once seemed possible were experiencing a return of malaria; in other places economic constraints forced premature relaxation of surveillance, and in some countries the control programs were curtailed because of political turmoil. There was evidence of widespread mosquito resistance to insecticides as well as reports of parasite resistance to the cheap and once effective antimalarial drugs, especially chloroquine and Fansidar. It was apparent to many public health scientists that the Global Eradication of Malaria Program was a failure and eradication could not be achieved. Clearly, a malaria vaccine was needed.

In 1956, Ian McGregor (1922–2007) and coworkers reported that newborn infants resident in The Gambia who had received weekly doses of the antimalarial drug chloroquine possessed significantly lower concentrations of γ-globulin than did a group of unprotected children.[54] A follow-up investigation using electrophoresis showed that although the γ-globulin concentration fell for the first 3–6 months after birth, subsequently there was a progressive rise with age similar to that of Europeans, but the level in the African children was always higher. These findings convinced McGregor there was an association of malaria with enhanced levels of serum γ-globulin, however at the time, there was no proof that the raised levels reflected a specific antibody response or that the γ-globulin response was protective and responsible for effective immunity. McGregor recognized that to conduct definitive experiments would require collaboration with an immunologist. He recruited Sydney Cohen (b. 1921) at Guy's Hospital in London to the project. When Cohen, an expert on γ-globulin, studied the synthesis of γ-globulin in Europeans and adult Gambians exposed to malaria, the former group was found to synthesize up to 80% less than the latter suggesting that the Gambians were making more γ-globulin as a protective response to malaria. McGregor arranged to collect a pool of serum from healthy Gambian volunteers and sent this to Cohen who carried out the fractionation. The 7S fraction of the γ-globulin from adult Gambian serum, judged to be pure by electrophoresis, as well as purified 7S γ-globulin fraction and serum minus the 7S fraction from adult Gambians was provided to McGregor. In addition, the 7S fraction from serum of UK blood donors was prepared as a control. Passive transfer experiments of immune serum were begun. Young Gambian children suffering from acute clinical *Plasmodium falciparum* and *P. malariae* as well as untreated children were injected intramuscularly at 8–24 hour intervals for three days with a total dose equivalent to 10–20% of a child's own γ-globulin. By the fourth day the parasite density did not increase and by the ninth day parasites were not seen in the blood in 8 out of 12 cases. Protection was limited, however, lasting only three months. Only the 7S fraction from immune adults reduced both the levels of parasites in the blood (asexual but not the sexual stages) and clinical illness. Here was the first reliable experimental data to support the view that humans repeatedly exposed to malaria-infected mosquitoes could develop an immunity capable of restricting clinical illness and parasite blood density, and that this immunity could be passively transferred to non-immunes (children) via γ-globulin.[55] These observations led to the proposal that, at least in theory, vaccination against malaria could be feasible. When McGregor and Cohen showed that the 7S fraction from adult Gambian serum had the same therapeutic effect in Tanzanian children with *P. falciparum,* it suggested that West and East African strains of malaria had immunological similarities and that a vaccine prepared against parasites from one region of Africa might be effective against parasites from other regions. This emboldened them (and others) to begin a hunt to identify the blood stage antigen responsible for protection against falciparum malaria.

In 1965 Cohen placed an advertisement in the *Observer* for a research assistant. Geoffrey Butcher (b. 1940), who had taken his B.Sc. at Kings College London (1962), was hired. At the time, the team (consisting of Cohen and Butcher!) at Guy's Hospital did not have access to human malaria parasites and so they began work with *P. knowlesi* as a surrogate for *P. falciparum.* At the outset, the idea was to repeat the experiments that Cohen and McGregor had carried out in The Gambia using passively transferred antibody, but this time using rhesus monkeys infected with minimal doses of *P. knowlesi* parasites. When it was discovered, however, that it took far too much antibody to get any effect in monkeys a test tube (*in vitro*) method was developed to assess protection.[56] Immune serum from animals challenged with a large parasite dose was tested on *P. knowlesi* in culture. The findings were interesting — immune serum had little influence on the growth of parasites within the red cell, but did inhibit merozoite invasion and eliminated the succeeding cycle of parasite development; this suggested that antibody combined with free merozoites to prevent re-invasion of red cells.[57] Now the pressing need was to identify the merozoite antigen(s).

In 1965 the WHO invited a group of scientists and health educators to its headquarters in Geneva to suggest innovative ways to rescue the failing Global Malaria Eradication Program. Paul Silverman (1924–2004) was an attendee.[58] Silverman served in the U.S. Army during World War II, received a bachelor's degree from Roosevelt University (Chicago) and completed an M.S. thesis on trypanosomes at Northwestern University (1950). Under the impression he was being rejected from admission to several medical schools because of membership in the Progressive Party (and had given the controversial Communist Paul Robeson a ride to an event) he moved to Israel where he began research on leishmaniasis under the direction of the eminent parasitologist Saul Adler. In 1953 Silverman moved to the UK and earned a Ph.D. in Parasitology and Epidemiology (1955) from the Liverpool School of Tropical Medicine for work on the identification of the mode of transmission of the beef tapeworm, showing that seagulls carried the infectious stages from sewage treatment outlets to meadows full of cows. Silverman's initial work on vaccination began at the Immunoparasitology Center of Allen and Hanburys Ltd (acquired in 1958 by GlaxoSmithKline (GSK)) in London, where he developed non-living vaccines to protect against tapeworm infections as well as round-worms of cattle, sheep, and horses. One vaccine, patented in 1959, described a non-living vaccine for the parasitic roundworms *Haemonchus* and *Trichinella* produced by *in vitro* incubation of third stage infective larvae, then removing these and freeze-drying the product excreted by the larvae (so-called exoantigens).

In the 1950s, Senator Joseph McCarthy launched a campaign to rid the U.S. of subversives who he claimed were strengthening communism and infiltrating government at all levels. As a consequence the American consulate suspended Silverman's passport until he named his "radical" friends from Chicago. Unable to travel he remained in the UK until there was a change in the U.S. political climate. With his travel privileges restored, Silverman, age 39, returned home to join the biological sciences faculty of the University of Illinois in Champaign–Urbana. His experience with non-living worm vaccines led him to propose that it would be possible to develop a protective vaccine against other parasitic infections, including malaria. Since sterile immunity, well documented in virus and bacterial infections, had not been observed with malaria parasites, Silverman's notion was contrary to the prevailing view of the majority of parasitologists and immunologists.

At the WHO meeting Silverman's proposal was for a vaccine that would target malaria transmission and pathology by a combination vaccine to two stages: the sporozoite and the asexual blood forms. At this time, there were formidable obstacles against achieving these goals. There was no laboratory method for continuously growing the blood stages of *P. falciparum* (or for that matter any other species infecting humans) for use in tests for protection, none of the human malarias had been adapted to infect primates, and there was no practical way to mass produce sporozoites of sufficient purity to be used as a vaccine. Silverman dismissed these hurdles as being "simply technical problems" that could be overcome by a major, well-funded research program. Several weeks later Silverman was invited to Washington, DC where he presented his plans to the Health Division of the United States Agency for International Development (USAID). USAID, having no in house scientific expertise, sent Silverman's proposal to an *ad hoc* panel of malaria researchers. Their judgment was, it was not feasible to develop a practical malaria vaccine for humans and consequently USAID should continue its business of distributing food and insecticides, providing advice, and assisting with economic programs and not invest in vaccine research. USAID ignored the expert advice and in 1966 elected to support a $1 million contract with the University of Illinois under the direction of Silverman. The project was designed to determine the feasibility of developing a vaccine against human malaria and involved testing of sporozoite and blood stage antigens and the *in vitro* cultivation of these stages.

When Silverman received the million-dollar USAID contract he began to recruit a team of researchers. I was one of the people he contacted. I visited with him at the University of Illinois and heard his plans. I was incredulous that he would consider developing a vaccine for human malaria since at the time there was no known way to produce large amounts of sporozoites or merozoites for use in vaccine trials. Further, were I to join Silverman's research group salary and research support would come from the 'soft' money provided by his two-year USAID contract. Because I already had a tenure track position and was supported by hard money at the University of California I turned down Silverman's offer, however there were others (Nelda Alger, Lawrence D'Antonio, Mary Barr, R. Schenkel and G. Simpson) who did sign on.

The USAID Malaria Immunology and Vaccine Research (MIVR) program began in 1966 under the aegis of project officer, Edgar A. Smith, a medical entomologist not an immunologist. In 1975, USAID sponsored a Workshop on *Problems Related to the Development of an Anti-malaria Vaccine* through the U.S. National Academy of Sciences to review the current status of research and to provide the agency with a more specific focus of approaches and priorities for development of a malaria vaccine. The panel of experts (including me) met in Albuquerque, NM. The panel proposed that USAID expand its support to several laboratories, and the means for increasing interest and cooperation among scientists in the area was discussed. Priorities were established: a continued emphasis on blood stage antigens including testing in monkeys, use of adjuvants, a continuation of basic studies of sporozoite immunization, and consideration of attenuated strains.

That same year in the UK, Cohen's group reported a spectacular finding: of six monkeys vaccinated twice intramuscularly with freshly isolated *P. knowlesi* merozoites emulsified in either Freund's complete adjuvant (FCA) or Freund's incomplete adjuvant (FIA) and challenged with the same variant no parasites were found in the blood in three and the remainder had a low grade infection (maximum 1.5%) that persisted for 6–11 days. Six other monkeys challenged with a variant different from the one used in vaccination with FCA showed a low-grade infection that terminated in less than two weeks. After initial challenge all surviving immunized animals were resistant to challenge for up to 16 weeks. Merozoite vaccination using FCA was required for resistance to challenge with a different variant but not for the same variant. Inoculation of blood from vaccinated animals after clearance of blood parasites into naïve monkeys did not result in an infection indicating that the vaccination had induced sterilizing immunity. Merozoites frozen in liquid nitrogen provided comparable protection, as did freeze-dried merozoites stored for up to 20 weeks at 4°C; the latter, however, gave somewhat less consistent protection. The work was hailed in a 1975 *British Medical Journal* article entitled "Malaria Vaccines on the Horizon."[59]

By the late 1970s, the claims and counterclaims of successful vaccination on both sides of the Atlantic, i.e. principally between the Cohen and Silverman groups led to questions as to whether the schizont or merozoite was better as an antigenic source. A competition was contemplated despite the fact that all of the previous vaccine trials required the toxic

FCA, the "pure" preparations still were not free of host cell contamination, the degree of protection was less than desirable for use in human trials, and in most cases the vaccinated animals became infected. At the time Cohen, the Chairman of the WHO Scientific Group on the Immunology of Malaria, was asked by USAID to visit New Mexico (where the Silverman USAID project had moved when he became Vice President for Research and Graduate Studies) to assess progress. It was suggested by a group of consultants (including myself) that to resolve the differences between the American and British vaccines there should be a direct comparison of the antigens in a single laboratory. At the time of this trial (1977) the USAID malaria vaccine program was under the direction of Karl Rieckmann, a physician, who had been taken on earlier by Silverman in the hope that he would conduct vaccine trials with human subjects. Without a suitable vaccine for humans, however, Rieckmann (now at the University of New Mexico) was to supervise a trial using rhesus monkeys, not human subjects. A total of 32 monkeys were used in the study. Eight controls and 24 rhesus monkeys were divided into groups of eight to test three antigenic materials from *P. knowlesi*: a frozen and thawed schizont preparation, a freeze-dried preparation, and fresh merozoites prepared by Sydney Cohen's associate Graham Mitchell at Guy's Hospital. Each preparation was emulsified in FCA, monkeys were inoculated intramuscularly twice at six-week intervals, and then they were challenged with a *P. knowlesi* variant different from the one used for vaccination. All controls developed severe blood infections and died within 12 days. Of those that received the frozen schizonts six died, while the surviving monkeys all had blood infections that lasted 10–14 days. Four of the eight monkeys that received the freeze-dried preparation died and the remaining animals had low-grade blood infections that persisted over a 9–15 day period; only two monkeys out of eight that had received the merozoite preparation survived. Clearly, none of the vaccine preparations was as successful as reported previously.

Silverman and Rieckmann blamed the poor showing of their vaccine on storage problems and countered that a fresh preparation might have produced better results, and the British claimed that, like good wine, their vaccine did not "travel well" and the prolonged period over which the merozoites were collected to obtain sufficient antigen for the second immunization may have contributed to the lower degree of protection. In a subsequent study a fresh merozoite preparation was prepared at Guy's Hospital, sent to the University of New Mexico in a frozen state, and then stored in liquid nitrogen until use; of eight monkeys vaccinated only four survived a challenge with blood parasites. The results of this head-to-head competition were presented at The Naval Medical Research Institute (NMRI)/USAID/WHO Workshop on the Immunology of Malaria held in Bethesda, MD on October 2–5, 1979. Upon peer review of these experiments the USAID contract to the University of New Mexico was terminated.

Despite these failures, immunization studies with the monkey malaria *P. knowlesi* did provide a background for a vaccine to protect against the human malaria, *P. falciparum*. In the 1960s, Quentin M. Geiman (1904–1986) at Stanford University (Palo Alto, CA) was encouraged by the U.S. Army Medical and Research Command, to cultivate *P. falciparum*. Despite his lack of recent experience with malaria, Geiman was the only one from the World War II Harvard University project who was available and interested in the cultivation of malaria parasites. However, unlike *P. knowlesi* (which Geiman had used at Harvard) he found it difficult to grow *P. falciparum in vitro*. Further, apart from nine cases of human malaria and two samples of infected blood there was no steady supply of falciparum parasites available in the San Francisco Bay Area and storage and freezing of blood caused changes in the parasite before *in vitro* culture began. Geiman tried to circumvent the shortage of human cases and investigated the possibility of adapting *P. falciparum* to New World *Aotus* (night owl) monkeys. Night owl monkeys obtained from a local dealer were given *P. falciparum*-infected blood from a soldier who had returned from Vietnam and later blood from a female patient who had contracted a *P. falciparum* infection in Uganda was used to infect a monkey. Infections were then transferred from these monkeys to other owl monkeys by inoculation of infected blood. At Stanford, the former line was named FVO, for Falciparum Vietnam Oak-Knoll and the latter FUP, for Falciparum Uganda Palo Alto.

To assist him in the cultivation of *P. falciparum*, Geiman recruited Wasim A.Siddiqui. Siddiqui had received a Ph.D. in 1961 from the

University of California at Berkeley working on amoebas, returned to India briefly, and then spent 1963–1966 working at the Rockefeller University with Trager studying the nutritional requirements of *P. lophurae.* At Stanford, and with support from a U.S. Army Department of Defense contract, Siddiqui used commercially available media for the short-term cultivation of *P. falciparum* in *Aotus* red blood cells ostensibly to produce high yields of malaria-infected red cells for isolation of antigens to be used in vaccination studies. In 1970, Geiman retired from Stanford University and shortly thereafter Siddiqui moved to the University of Hawaii.

The successful culture of *P. falciparum* by Trager and Jensen in 1976 encouraged USAID to advertise for additional contractors to improve on the cultivation of the red blood cell stages of malaria, culturing different strains, developing methods to produce gametocytes, and to provide methods for harvesting parasite antigens and testing their immune potential. There were 25 responses and "after intensive review" 10 projects in the so-called "collaborating network" including the University of Hawaii were funded.

The USAID contract with the University of Hawaii (Principal Investigator Wasim Siddiqui) was dedicated to developing a malaria vaccine and continuing to improve on methods for *in vitro* cultivation of *P. falciparum.* Siddiqui and coworkers extended the earlier immunization studies of rhesus monkeys to *Aotus* by attempting to vaccinate against *P. falciparum.* Taking clues from the knowlesi studies they used a merozoite-enriched preparation from short-term *in vitro* cultures of *Aotus* infected with *P. falciparum* (FUP). Two doses of vaccine (2.73 mg total protein) emulsified with FCA were administered intramuscularly at three-week intervals and three weeks following the second vaccination the animals were challenged by intravenous injection of blood containing 600,000 parasites. All the control animals died within two weeks with fulminating infections whereas three of the vaccinated monkeys survived, however, all had low-grade blood infections.[60]

Siddiqui recognized that a barrier to the development of a protective malaria vaccine was the need for a suitable replacement for FCA. He wrote: "the ultimate objective of all malaria vaccine studies is to develop a vaccine that can be used to immunize and protect man, not monkeys or rodents.

Therefore the development of an immunologically satisfactory and pharmacologically acceptable adjuvant is imperative in the development of a malaria vaccine acceptable for use in man."[61] Siddiqui's group tried muramyl dipeptide (MDP), a substance reportedly able to replace whole tubercle bacteria in FCA, and which had already been shown to enhance the immunological response of animals against an antigen when injected with FIA (mineral oil). However, vaccination trials of *Aotus* with merozoites in MDP in peanut oil or mineral oil were unsuccessful.

Siddiqui and coworkers continued to pursue alternatives to FCA. They tried stearoyl-MDP adjuvant with carrier liposomes (cholesterol plus lecithin). The vaccine contained a crude antigen of infected blood containing 50–60% schizonts with merozoites and the reminder other developmental stages (2.86 mg total protein) emulsified in the adjuvant. Animals were vaccinated twice at four-week intervals and 17 days after the last dose the monkeys were challenged with 750,000 parasites (FUP) obtained from an ongoing blood infection in an *Aotus* monkey. Two of the controls died within two weeks of challenge and remarkably the third control despite having 25% of its red cells infected survived. All four of the immunized monkeys survived challenge, two developing low-grade infections that lasted a week, two developed infections ranging from 5–15%. A limited number of owl monkeys became negative for blood parasites after a month, however, since blood from these animals was not injected into naïve monkeys it was not known whether the animals still harbored small numbers of parasites undetectable by microscopy. The results, reported in a *Science* article titled: "Vaccination of experimental monkeys against *P. falciparum*. A possible safe adjuvant," was considered to be important and significant (especially by Siddiqui and USAID) since the stearoyl-MDP adjuvant and liposomes did not produce an inflammatory reaction at the injection site (as would Freund's complete adjuvant) and claimed "an effective, safe malaria vaccine may be possible."[60]

Siddiqui's group also immunized *Aotus* monkeys with a crude merozoite preparation that he considered to be a vaccine. This vaccine could not be used with human subjects, however, despite this limitation USAID publicized the findings as if a human subject vaccination trial was surely in the near future. Press conferences were called, the State of Hawaii legislature expressed gratitude to Siddiqui and the University of Hawaii honored him with its most prestigious award for excellence in research stating this was for his "finding the first promising candidate for a malaria vaccine." There were further exaggerated claims: he was the first to culture malaria parasites and the first to infect owl monkeys with human malaria. USAID was also wildly enthusiastic: "technically speaking a vaccine may be available for human testing as early as 1985."[62] In reality, there was no vaccine to be tested in humans.

In 1982, Smith, the Project Office for the USAID MIVR Program, retired and was succeeded by James M. Erickson, an economic entomologist with a Ph.D. in population ecology from Cornell University. Erickson was, as his predecessor, without experience in vaccine development. Under Erickson a stubborn, abrasive, fast-talking, and irreverent malaria vaccine booster the MIVR that had been funded at less than $4 million per annum would grow substantially and by 1988 the malaria program's budget was $8.5 million (NY Times July 17, 1988).

With Erickson at the helm USAID decided that a large number of candidate vaccines suitable for testing in humans would be available and it was believed that before this could occur they would have to be tested in South American owl (*Aotus*) and squirrel (*Saimiri*) monkeys from Peru, Colombia, and Bolivia to measure the toxicity of the vaccine, possible harmful effects and ability to protect against malaria. In 1982 USAID awarded a three-year subcontract to the Malaria Institute in Colombia with an estimated budget of $709,375 and two months later American Institute of Biological Sciences (AIBS, a respectable non-profit group that had managed various biological and biomedical projects for the federal government) was asked by USAID to amend the contract and increase the funding to $1.53 million to cover AIBS overhead and research costs. The Principal Investigator for the Colombian program was Carlos Espinal. Although there were research components to the program the primary motive for the contract was to obtain Colombian monkeys. By 1984 an AIBS audit found numerous billing and financial irregularities at the Malaria Institute. Three sets of books were found. Espinal was unable to account for all project funds and the U.S. dollar checks mailed by AIBS to the malaria unit had been converted into local currency "through channels forbidden by national monetary authorities." Further, some 40 checks valued at ~$150,000 made out to the Colombian Malaria Institute were deposited in Swiss banks and other accounts outside Colombia. AIBS alleged that Espinal defrauded the U.S. government and a U.S. District Court indicted him for the crime. The Malaria Institute suspended its malaria activities; no further work was performed during the remainder of the contract period and nothing more was heard from Espinal. USAID did not seek to recover any expenses from AIBS or the Malaria Institute due to "sensitive relations" between the U.S. and Colombia.[63]

In April 1985, USAID decided to purchase up to 600 Bolivian monkeys using unexpended funds from the suspended AIBS subcontract with the Colombian National Institutes of Health. AIBS, the management arm of the vaccine program was to arrange for the purchase of the monkeys and a person named George Diaz would be given a contract to find and acquire the monkeys. Diaz and Erickson then contacted Worldwide Primates based in Miami, FL to obtain 200 owl monkeys at $475 each and 400 squirrel monkeys at $375 each for a total of $245,000. Diaz then told AIBS that the monkeys would be obtained from Gerrick International for $336,000–$630 for each *Aotus* and $520 for each *Saimiri*. It turned out that Gerrick International was a shell corporation for Diaz and Erickson. On September 12, 1985, Erickson had ordered stationery with the letterhead Gerrick International and Diaz opened a bank account in the name of Gerrick International. AIBS issued a check for $168,000 to Gerrick International in partial payment for monkeys and Gerrick in turn paid Worldwide Primates $122,500. In October 1985 Gerrick was paid the remainder of the $168,000 and presumably Erickson and Diaz made a profit on this also. In January 1986 Diaz wrote a check for $8,500 to his brother-in-law and this was then signed over to Erickson. In March, $11,886 was withdrawn from the Gerrick account and the money was used to purchase two cashier's checks made payable to J. Erickson.[63]

Erickson might have escaped without punishment had it not been for the continuing probe by the Inspector General and the General Accounting Office (GAO) into procurement of monkeys and Gerrick International. A grand jury used this to level charges against Erickson of conspiracy, conflict of interest, and accepting a gratuity. Since he paid no tax on the profits from Gerrick International Erickson was indicted on three counts of submitting false tax returns.[63] In 1990 after pleading guilty a lenient court sentenced him to six months, to be served in a halfway house, and fined him $20,000. He served his time and was not heard from again.

Wasim Siddiqui at the University of Hawaii also became entangled in the web of misappropriation of funds associated with the USAID malaria vaccine program. As noted earlier Siddiqui's group had immunized *Aotus* monkeys with a crude vaccine made from cultured *P. falciparum* mixed with FCA and although a few of the vaccinated monkeys were protected from challenge all had low numbers of parasites in the blood. In 1984, Siddiqui submitted a proposal to USAID to extend his research for another three years at a cost of $1.65 million. USAID sent the proposal to two external reviewers. Reviewer 1 wrote, "The proposal is mediocre, overly ambitious and the budget is overwhelming and excessive" and the second reviewer (me) said, "the proposal is unrealistic in terms of time, money and availability of material. The amount of money requested is outlandish and outrageous." Yet Siddiqui received his funding and by 1986 Siddiqui would write 'the asexual blood stage vaccine may soon be available for clinical trial.'"[62]

In 1988, acting on 'information received" the Office of Inspector General (OIG) of USAID began investigating Siddiqui's and the University of Hawaii's handling of research funds.[63] The OIG reported that there was evidence to support the allegations that the Principal Investigator (Siddiqui) apparently diverted funds to himself and his secretary's personal use and (monies) were used to refurbish his offices at the University and these construction costs were charged to the grant as consultant payments. On September 14, 1989, the Grand Jury in Hawaii indicted Siddiqui and his administrative assistant Susan Lofton with theft in the third degree and criminal conspiracy. The Deputy Attorney General of Hawaii charged that some of the USAID money was siphoned off between 1984 and 1987 through illicit accounting tricks and a kickback arrangement with a Honolulu travel agency that Siddiqui had engaged to run a 1985 Asia Pacific Conference on Malaria. The USAID conference check was deposited with the Research Corporation of the University of Hawaii and at Siddiqui's direction was to pay the bills for the conference. There was $100,000 as an advance payment for services to be used as a deposit to the Pacific Hotel where the conference was to be held. In March 1985, a month before the conference Siddiqui instructed the travel agency to begin paying him directly $1,260 per month and to pay his secretary $1,000 a month. These salary supplements were to continue for the next two years. Between December 1984 and April 1986 the travel agency paid Siddiqui $17,400 and Lofton $16,000. USAID was sent a bill for $35,425 for services and departmental rental related to the conference. USAID paid the bill, but the indictment disputes that the money was used for that purpose.[64] This was only the beginning of USAID's troubles. Hawaii's Senator Daniel K. Inouye, Chairman of the Senate Appropriations Committee on Foreign Operations, which has jurisdiction over the USAID budget launched a GAO investigation of the entire $8.5 million malaria vaccine program budget. The October 18, 1989, Washington Post reported[65] that the GAO had found irregularities at the University of Hawaii and as a result Siddiqui and his Administrative Assistant were indicted of stealing USAID research contract monies. By chance, the indictment came out the same day the University of Hawaii received word that USAID had renewed Siddiqui's contract for three years (worth $1.65 million). However, the USAID insisted that Siddiqui be removed from the project until the charges were resolved. Legal maneuvering continued for years, but it finally ended in 1993 when Siddiqui pleaded no contest to embezzlement charges and was sentenced to six months of house detention.[66] The University of Hawaii relieved Siddiqui of teaching duties, however, he continued to report to the campus wearing a court-ordered radio bracelet to alert police to his where-abouts. The University professors' union successfully defended Siddiqui's assertion that he not be dismissed because there was no just cause and he did not lose his retirement pension. On the day he retired Siddiqui pleaded no contest to a civil suit brought against him for $250,000.[67,68]

Along with Erickson and Siddiqui the reputations of other scientists were damaged and funding of USAID supported research programs was reduced albeit temporarily. In 1987–1988 after USAID sent onsite review teams to the Agouron Institute (Reese project) and to the Biomedical Research Institute in Rockville Maryland (BRI), where Michael Hollingdale had a contract to develop culture systems for EE stages of *P. vivax* and *P. falciparum* and to characterize the liver receptor for the sporozoite and Werner Zolg was to develop a DNA vaccine for blood stages, both contracts were terminated. At some institutions there were complaints of a lack of objectivity by the review team as well as incomplete disclosure of research findings lest data be given away to reviewers with a competing interest; one of the institutions reviewed stated that a member of the review team was prejudiced and had submitted a proposal for funding knowing this would depend on availability of funds in a very restricted budget environment, and another member of the review team was accused of "pursuing precisely an identical line of research to ours." These objections were rejected by USAID. In 1988 the project on antigen localization and to assess purity of blood-stage antigen preparations, and to determine the structure and function of knobs, headed by Susan Langreth of the Uniformed Services University of the Health Sciences in Bethesda, MD, and rumored to be Erickson's paramour, was terminated without any review. Leveling a complaint she claimed she had been threatened with repossession of an electron microscope that had been purchased under her USAID contract. The claim was denied.

The conclusion of the 1989 GAO report was that in the MIVR there was evidence of fraud and waste of government funds, that subprojects were selected under questionable circumstances, performance was not subject to adequate evaluation and poor quality research may have been tolerated. To correct such deficiencies USAID appointed a new management group (Atlantic Resources Inc.) with Carter Diggs, formerly director of the Army's malaria vaccine program, as a scientific consultant. Under his leadership there was an improvement in the evaluation of subprojects using an expanded list of consultants to review proposals and an insistence on high-quality proposals from institutions seeking funding.

In 1992 USAID elected to shift emphasis from support of research to development of promising vaccine candidates and to testing of investigational vaccines. USAID formed the Malaria Vaccine Development Program (MVDP) effectively replacing the MIVR to build a pipeline from early preclinical vaccine development, through the regulatory process and field-testing of vaccine candidates. The most advanced blood stage vaccine, the merozoite surface protein (FMP1/AS02A), developed on the initiative of USAID at Walter Reed Army Institute of Research (WRAIR) with GSK, was the culmination of work begun in 1995 and until 2000 major operating expenses were borne by USAID. Since 2006 the USAID budget for malaria vaccines has been effectively leveraged through a pooling of resources by partners such as Program for Appropriate Technology in Health (PATH), Malaria Vaccine Initiative (MVI), GSK, WRAIR, and NMRI.

Chapter 6
Dreaming of a Nobel Prize

William Trager, during the time I was with him in his Rockefeller Institute laboratory as a post-doctoral fellow, lacked airs of self-importance. He was a bench scientist, dedicated and meticulous in both the design and conduct of his experiments. I remember seeing him day after day, peering through his wire-rimmed glasses at stained slides under the microscope, or with sleeves of his shirt rolled up, bent over a Bunsen burner flame transferring cultures. He prepared his own media and recorded each day's results in a bound notebook in an unmistakable and an almost illegible handwriting. During a span of 40 years he devoted all of his efforts toward an understanding of the nutritional requirements of *Plasmodium* and he cared not one whit for vaccines. But by 1979 his attitude had changed. More and more (or so it appeared to me) he became convinced that he could prepare a vaccine from his blood cultures of *Plasmodium falciparum*.

Trager was acutely aware of the seminal discoveries made in the 1940s at the Harvard Medical School and that this work had led to a shared 1954 Nobel Prize for John Enders, Frederick Robbins and Thomas Weller.[69] And, Trager who was a contemporary of the driven, curious, and dedicated microbe hunter, Weller, knew him well. Thomas Weller (1915–2008), as an undergraduate at the University of Michigan had spent two summers under the well-respected parasitologists L. J. Thomas and W. W. Cort at the University of Michigan Biological Station and had described a roundworm that parasitized perch. Upon completion of the A.B. degree he intended to study parasites at the Harvard Medical School, however, after taking a

93

microbiology course taught by Hans Zinsser (an expert on typhus and author of the classic *Rats, Lice, and History*) his interest in microbes was piqued. However, he did not give up on parasites altogether and one summer as a medical student Weller went to Florida to study malaria at a Rockefeller Foundation training center. During his time at Harvard University Weller visited the Rockefeller Institute in New York City and was exposed to the methods for growing viruses using chick embryo tissue cultures. In his fourth year of medical school Weller wanted to see whether the larval stages of the roundworm *Trichinella* found in muscle could mature into adults in the presence of living tissue cells and so he began a tutorial project with Enders, an associate of Zinsser, who had earlier turned from the study of bacterial immunity to investigations on the growth of viruses using roller tube cultures. Shortly after Weller received his M.D. (1940) his clinical training was interrupted by the outbreak of World War II and military service. The U.S. Army Medical Corps sent Weller to Puerto Rico where he focused on the diagnosis and control of malaria. The U.S. Army Sanitary Corps posted Trager to New Guinea where he worked on malaria control through atabrine treatment. At War's end both returned to their respective academic institutions — Weller to Harvard and Trager to Rockefeller.

Weller had carried out a crucial experiment almost by chance.[69] Using chopped up animal tissues such as placenta, brain, and kidney it was possible to grow the cells in laboratory flasks as a single layer. This was called tissue culture. After inoculating 16 tissue culture flasks with the throat washings from a child suffering from chicken pox. Weller had four flasks left over and he thought it would be interesting to inoculate these with a mouse brain suspension that contained poliovirus. The chicken pox virus did not grow but the fluid from the poliovirus did and in the process the tissue culture cells were destroyed. Subsequently, Weller and Robbins found that the fluids from the tissue grown poliovirus would paralyze mice and monkeys. Mixing infected fluid with antibodies to the virus prevented growth of the virus in the tissue cultures and monkeys were protected from paralysis. In Weller's hands and with improvements in tissue culture methods different antigenic types of the poliovirus were isolated from fecal samples. These could be grown in laboratory flasks and characterized. Finally, Enders, Robbins, and Weller were able to show — as had Louis

Pasteur 75 years earlier — that multiple passages in tissue culture decreased the virulence of the poliovirus. This attenuation of the poliovirus would ultimately lead to a live protective vaccine against polio.

Trager found comfort in the words Weller had spoken in his Nobel lecture: "tissue culture in some form might eventually prove of value in developing a prophylactic agent ... (and) immunizing materials ... through the use of *in vitro* techniques is already more than a theoretical possibility."[69] It was after Trager's feat of "taming" falciparum had been achieved that he began to think more and more of Weller's serendipitous discovery and felt his success with culture of *P. falciparum* was similar to Weller's poliovirus work. Perhaps when there was a malaria vaccine for which a Nobel Prize would be awarded, Trager might have mused, he might also be considered for such recognition.

The stated objective of the 1977 WHO-sponsored Workshop on the *Biology and In Vitro Cultivation of Malaria Parasites* was "to review the status of research and to identify areas in which progress were most needed to further expansion of chemotherapeutic and immunologic research." The venue for the workshop was the campus of Rockefeller University, and it was a celebration of the achievement of Trager and Jensen. As Trager walked across the Rockefeller campus, he announced to several of those within earshot, "You know, using *in vitro* cultures, there will be a protective malaria vaccine in five years." I was astounded at his declaration, and brashly countered, "You cannot be serious; it will be decades, if ever, before there is a practical vaccine." However, he was serious, as was another who walked with us, an immunologist, Ruth Nussenzweig, who put a finger across her lips, saying, "Shush. We must promise a malaria vaccine is on the horizon or else research funding will quickly dry up."

In 1978, when Trager obtained research funds from United States Agency for International Development (USAID) he recruited a team to carry out vaccine research: Robert Reese an immunologist would study the protection afforded by the isolated antigens. Susan Langreth, an electron microscopist, would monitor the purity of the isolated antigenic fractions. Harold Stanley's expertise in tissue culture would be used to improve the *in vitro* culture conditions and Araxie Kilejian, a biochemist, was to isolate and purify antigens. To support the USAID-sponsored program Trager was given a large budget, and a number of laboratory rooms to accommodate the increased number of investigators. Schizonts and mature trophozoites, harvested from Trager–Jensen cultures of *P. falciparum* (FCR-3 strain), were used to prepare merozoites by saponin lysis and this served as the vaccine. The first experiment employed six monkeys: three received merozoites emulsified in Freund's complete antigen (FCA) administered intramuscularly and a booster vaccination was given three weeks later consisting of the same number of merozoites however this time emulsified in Freund's incomplete adjuvant (FIA). The three controls received only an injection of the adjuvant. (A more suitable control would have been uninfected red cells, however, that was not done). Three weeks after the second vaccination the animals were challenged by intravenous inoculation of one million parasitized red cells of the same strain derived from an *Aotus* monkey. Within 2–3 weeks after being challenged all of the monkeys were dead with blood infections ranging from 10–55%.[70]

In the belief that the amount of antigen was more important than the manner of administration the protocol was altered so that three intramuscular injections were given at three-week intervals, with the first two containing merozoite antigen emulsified with muramyl dipeptide (MDP a synthetic derivative of N-acetylmuramyl-L-alanyl-D-isoglutamine) and mineral oil (FIA), and the third solely the antigen in mineral oil.[70] (The basis for using MDP was that Graham Mitchell, working in Cohen's group at Guy's Hospital, found MDP to have some protective effect, i.e. two out of six monkeys survived challenge when vaccinated with merozoite antigen emulsified in MDP and FIA.[71,72] This result was in contrast to FCA, where five out of six vaccinated animals survived challenge.) Although the number of merozoites in the vaccine given to each monkey had been increased and the challenge injection reduced to 500,000 infected red blood cells, two out of three vaccinated monkeys died. One died a week later than controls, a second died two weeks after the controls, and the surviving third monkey had a low-grade infection. All of the "protected" *Aotus* monkeys showed anemia and in those that succumbed this was assumed to be the cause.

Reese and colleagues claimed the work to be "significant for two major reasons": merozoites from *P. falciparum* cultured *in vitro* for over a year were still able to induce immunity, that is they had not lost their antigenic "punch" and synthetic MDP could substitute for FCA when a sufficient amount of antigen was used.[70] Subsequent studies at Rockefeller University reported on the inhibitory effects of immune serum on *in vitro* growth[73] of *P. falciparum* where inhibition was claimed to be due to the reaction with surface alterations (called knobs) on the falciparum infected red blood cell, not merozoites!

In 1980, Reese, wanting to get out from being under Trager's shadow, moved his laboratory and several of his Rockefeller University colleagues across the country to the Scripps Research Institute (La Jolla, CA). At Scripps, where immunology was in the forefront, Reese was joined by Randall Howard and Harold Stanley and together they studied the synthesis of merozoite proteins,[74] developed an assay for measuring the effects of immune sera on *in vitro* parasite maturation,[75] prepared antibodies from *Aotus* monkeys and used these to identify a merozoite surface antigen,[76] constructed a cDNA library and screened this with serum from immune *Aotus* to identify three merozoite surface antigens[77,78] one of which was related to so-called heat shock proteins. When Reese did not gain tenure at Scripps the USAID project was moved to the Agouron Institute (also in La Jolla, CA). There the Reese laboratory carried out immunological modeling and peptide mapping and antibody responses to the heat shock protein. However, for the most part these "significant finds" produced nothing of any importance toward the development of a protective malaria vaccine for humans. Indeed, in 1987, after a negative review of the project by a group of scientific consultants (of which I was one), the USAID contract to the Agouron Institute was terminated. Shortly thereafter, Reese and his collaborators left the field of malaria vaccine research.

The USAID malaria vaccine program illustrates the problem with so-called push programs i.e. those that pay for research inputs rather than results and where funds are committed before a product is developed. In push programs applicants tend to exaggerate the prospects that their approach will succeed and once funded researchers may divert the resources to other products and to pursue avenues that will more rapidly advance their careers. Indeed, even when it was clear that there were problems in finding a protective malaria vaccine using monkey models researchers kept requesting more funding and USAID administrators kept approving it. This resulted, in part, from researchers tending to look favorably on the promise of their own work (the Pygmalion effect) and administrators having the incentive to expand their own programs (the Emperor effect). In the development of a malaria vaccine the perils inherent in push programs must be recognized and avoided.

　　To its credit USAID was one of the first agencies to recognize the need for a malaria vaccine and it funded such research when others had either ignored or abandoned responsibility. However, those who were responsible for the USAID Malaria and Immunology and Vaccine Research Program were neither patient nor realistic, and they did not want to countenance the fact that vaccine development can be a slow and deliberate process. Seeking to ensure that funds would continue to be provided USAID and the network contractors did not produce a realistic timetable of 15 or 20 years or perhaps longer — something they feared the public and government would not like to hear — and so they promised a "magic bullet" in just a few years. The significance of the vaccination results were frequently exaggerated and given undue prominence. Within USAID there was a lack of critical self-assessment and accountability, a disregard of the advice of professionals, and an unbridled desire to be the first developer of a protective vaccine. The malaria investigators sponsored by USAID became an exclusive club whose members were its cheerleaders. Because of a fear of loss of funding members in the USAID Malaria and Immunology Vaccine Research Program never expressed dissent and the critical comments by reviewers (including myself as a consultant to the USAID MIVR Program from 1983–1991) were rarely heeded.

Chapter 7

Molecular Biology Assists in Vaccine Development

DNA is the stuff of which genes are made. Each DNA molecule is made up of building blocks called nucleotides, and in turn, each is made up of three major constituents: (1) phosphate, (2) a sugar, deoxyribose, and (3) a base. The phosphate and sugar are constant features, but the bases come in four varieties: the double-ringed purines, adenine (A), guanine (G) and the single-ringed pyrimidines, thymine (T), and cytosine (C). The percentage of purines equals that of pyrimidines; in a shorthand way A = T and G = C, and A + G = T + C. In 1953, Maurice Wilkins, James Watson, and Francis Crick using this information and the results of Rosalind Franklin's X-ray crystallographic work[a] were able to build a structural model that solved how the bases and sugar and phosphate were arranged. It was a ladder-like molecule with two long chains of sugar-phosphate forming the uprights and the bases — a purine pairing with a pyrimidine — linking the two uprights, as would the rungs of a ladder. According to the pattern of the X-ray the two strands of DNA were twisted around one another in the form of a helix (similar to a spiral staircase). They called it a double helix. In 1962 Watson, Crick, and Wilkins shared the Nobel Prize in Physiology or Medicine. (Rosalind Franklin whose crystallographic work was critical

---

[a]In X-ray crystallography X-rays are shot at a crystal of material and the scattering recorded on a photographic plate reveals the three dimensional form of that material.

to understanding the structure of DNA had died in 1958 from ovarian cancer and hence was ineligible to share in the prize.)

The Watson–Crick model of DNA provides a basis for the molecule to duplicate itself. One strand of the DNA is complementary to the other since when an A occurs in one strand a T occurs on the opposite stand, and when there is a G on one strand this is paired with a C in the other strand. The strands are able to separate by the paired nitrogenous bases moving apart; this "unzipping" of the strands allows a complementary strand to be formed from nucleotides and other molecules in the cell, under the direction of an enzyme, DNA polymerase. All the information necessary for arranging the bases in a linear sequence to complement the original strands of DNA is provided for by the mechanism of complementary base pairing. For example, if one strand contains A then a T nucleotide will pair with it, and if the next base is a G then a C will pair with it. In this manner the old strands of DNA direct the sequence or order of the nucleotides in the new sister strands. The new strand is a complementary copy of the original strand, and the two new strands are identical to the original; importantly because of complementary base pairing the exact sequence in the original double helix will be faithfully reproduced. This process is called DNA duplication or replication. A particular sequence of bases in the DNA comprises a gene, and that particular sequence codes for the specific product, a protein, consisting of a string of amino acids. The genetic code is "written" as a three-letter code because each "word" is composed of a three (triplet) base sequence. Each triplet codes for a single amino acid. For example, the three letter sequence CGA, CGG, CGT, and CGC code for the amino acid alanine.

The differences between living things — be they human or *Plasmodium* — is not that they have different nucleotides in their DNA but is due to the differences in the sequential order of the bases. It is much like using the letters in the alphabet to make different words. The letters used may be the same, however, the words formed and their meaning (message) can differ depending on the way the letters are arranged.

The genetic code in the DNA molecule is like a set of blueprints housed in a library, but the blueprints cannot leave the library (nucleus). Consequently, in order to direct the manufacture of the gene product (protein) there is blueprint transcriber as well as a translator of the code, the molecules messenger

RNA (mRNA), and transfer RNA (tRNA) respectively. These RNAs also contain four nitrogenous bases but instead of T there is uracil (U), the sugar is ribose not deoxyribose, and the molecules are not in the form of a double helix but are single strands. When a gene is to be transcribed (copied) the DNA double helix unzips and a faithful copy using complementary base pairing is made into mRNA by means of an enzyme, RNA polymerase. The mRNA leaves the library (nucleus) and moves to the cytoplasm where it attaches to an RNA-containing particle, the ribosome. At the ribosome the mRNA is translated into a protein. Each amino acid, corresponding to an mRNA triplet is ferried by means of a tRNA of which there are 20 different ones for each of 20 amino acids. The ribosome acts like a jig to hold the mRNA in place and guides the tRNA-amino acid into proper alignment for coupling. As the ribosome moves along the strand of mRNA "reading" the message a string of amino acids (= protein) is formed. This process is called translation. In short, genetic information flows: DNA- → RNA- → protein.

A change in the sequence of DNA either by deletion of a base or by the substitution of a different base may lead to a change in the mRNA sequence and in turn to a different sequence of amino acids and hence a different protein. Such a genetic change — a mutation — may result in either a meaningful message or a meaningless one.

In the early 1970s, recombinant DNA technology made possible the isolation of genes from a variety of sources. The recombinant DNA method (as originally developed) used plasmids — small circles of naked DNA. Both strands of a circular plasmid double helix could be severed at a specific location with molecular scissors known as restriction enzymes. When mixed in the same test tube with a second DNA (such as *Plasmodium* DNA) that had been similarly cleaved, and in the presence of another enzyme (called ligase), the snipped ends could be "glued" together; the end result was the creation of a hybrid or recombinant plasmid. These mixtures of DNA could then be used to infect bacteria. After bacterial growth in a Petri dish containing antibiotics, only the recombinant DNA plasmids would enable the bacteria to survive. In some instances, the bacteria containing the recombinant plasmid would express the protein encoded by the foreign DNA. Although plasmid based vectors were used early on, later it was found that engineered viruses called bacteriophage were more efficient vectors and the number of clones generated was greater than that found for plasmids. In addition, handling of large numbers of phage and screening of recombinant clones was far easier.

Gene expression libraries can be constructed using genomic DNA. These expression libraries are often constructed from sheared DNA or DNA partially digested with nuclease, including restriction enzymes, able to chop up the DNA into small pieces. To be able to handle these pieces of DNA it is necessary to copy and store them, just as a book needs to be printed and bound. In the copying process, each fragment of DNA is attached to the DNA of a bacteriophage. After the DNA of the malaria parasite has been chopped up into small pieces of DNA and attached to phage DNA, the phage can be used to infect the bacterium *E. coli*. Each phage carries its own DNA as well as fragments of malaria parasite DNA. When the surface of a Petri dish is covered with a lawn of *E. coli* infected with such a phage clear spots appear on the bacterial lawn where the viruses have killed (lysed) the bacteria. These spots, called plaques, contain millions of virus particles with millions of copies of the original pieces of malarial DNA. Theoretically, genomic libraries have all the DNA sequences present at equal frequency.

Another kind of library, a complementary DNA (cDNA) expression library, is somewhat more difficult to prepare because it first requires the isolation of the transitory and unstable mRNA; however, in this library the sequences are present in proportion to their abundance as mRNA molecules and thus represent differentially expressed genes. In other words, the mRNA is a concise working copy of the DNA code. The mRNA can be faithfully copied into a stable and complementary form, called cDNA, using the enzyme, reverse transcriptase. As with the method for producing a genomic DNA library when the cDNA is inserted into a plasmid or a phage and the *E. coli* infected the DNA is copied and in some instances it is possible to have a protein product.

Powerful as the recombinant DNA methods are, there is a significant limitation: it requires growing large volumes of bacteria to amplify the DNA of interest as well as a considerable investment in time and research funds to identify the recombinant clones of interest. By 1985 it was largely replaced by the polymerase chain reaction (PCR), a technique called "molecular photocopying." In brief: two short stretches of single stranded DNA (called primers), corresponding in nitrogenous base sequence to the regions bracketing a DNA expanse of interest, such as a specific gene, are synthesized. The primers are added to the DNA template, i.e. total genomic DNA or a cDNA population of interest, and the DNA is "melted" by heating to 90–95°C to separate the helical strands. Upon cooling, the primer can bind to its complementary stretch of single stranded template DNA. In addition, present in the test tube is an enzyme, DNA polymerase, and all four bases. The polymerase will only begin incorporating bases where the DNA is already double stranded, and so it begins adding bases at the end of the primer and synthesizes the DNA region that follows. By using a thermal cycler, one that heats ("melts") and cools ("anneals"), the process can be repeated every five minutes and the stretch of DNA of interest will copied again and again; in two hours the DNA of interest will be increased about 34 million-fold. This amplified DNA can then be sequenced (= read).

In the sequencing method developed by Frederick Sanger the strands of DNA are duplicated by means of DNA polymerase in the presence of a mixture of the normal nucleotides A, T, G, C plus some dideoxy A (ddA) or ddT, or ddG or ddC. If the polymerase incorporates the normal base the DNA chain grows but when it encounters a dideoxynucleotide it stops lengthening. The result is four different samples, each containing a series of DNA chains of varying length depending where in the growing chain the different dideoxynucleotides were incorporated opposite the complementary T, A, C, or G template bases during the replication process. Each sample is placed on a gel and the fragments separated by electrophoresis: short chains move faster and longer chains slower. The positions can be read off such that the shortest fragment will contain the first base, the next larger the second and so on. Later, this four-lane method of manual sequencing was replaced by one that could automatically read out the order of bases in a stretch of DNA using a single lane: a different colored dye for each type of chain terminating dideoxynucleotide was added to the polymerase mix and incubated. By subjecting the single lane sample to an electric field all the DNA pieces can be sorted according to size. With ultraviolet light illumination each fragment fluoresces differently depending on its terminal dideoxynucleotide; by scanning the fluorescent pattern and feeding this into a computer the base sequence of a gene or a piece of a gene can be printed out.

Craig Venter (b. 1946) has been described by his critics as an egotistical, narcissistic, and ruthless entrepreneur bent on making billions of dollars from sequencing genomes and by his supporters as a passionate, brilliant visionary who tamed the power of genomics to radically transform healthcare by sequencing the human genome.[79] Venter received his B.S. in Biochemistry from UC San Diego in 1972 and his Ph.D. in Physiology and Pharmacology from the same institution in 1975. He worked for a short time at SUNY Buffalo and then in 1984 Venter joined the NIH where he learned the technique of rapidly identifying all the mRNAs present in a cell using short cDNA sequence fragments called expressed sequence tags (ESTs).

An EST is produced by one-shot sequencing of several hundred base pairs from an end of a cDNA clone taken from a cDNA library. These clones consist of DNA that is complementary to mRNA, hence the ESTs represent portions of expressed genes. ESTs can be mapped to specific chromosome locations and, if the genome of the organism that originated the EST has been sequenced one can align the EST sequence to that genome.

Originally, the use of ESTs was controversial since most geneticists felt it would not be accurate enough to sequence an entire organism. Unhappy with the support of NIH Venter left in 1992 to establish The Institute for Genomic Research (TIGR) dedicated to using the shotgun technique for the sequencing of a variety of microbes. In a few short years Venter's 'whole genome shotgun sequencing approach' was successfully used to sequence the bacterial genomes of *Haemophilus influenzae*, *Mycoplasma genitalae*, and *Borrelia burgdorfi* the causative agent of Lyme disease.

As early as 1994, frustrated with the slow progress and inefficient use of labor on the publicly funded Human Genome Project (begun in 1990), and unable to get his own funding, Venter decided the same approach could be used to sequence the human genome. In 1998, Venter left TIGR to become the first President of Celera Genomics (a company established by Perkin Elmer for the purpose of generating and commercializing genomic information and to use their automated sequencing machines). One year later, his team at Celera applied the shotgun approach to the *Drosophila* genome as a proof of principle and then to the human genome using 300

DNA sequencers, a powerful computer, and a technique developed by Gene Meyers, a mathematician (from the University of Arizona and recruited to Celera) for reassembling the sequences from the shotgun approach. Meyer's algorithms which allowed the fragments of DNA to be aligned and 'stitched' together was scorned by his scientific peers for being error-prone and unworkable, but at Celera he proved the technique could work. Two years later, the race to sequence the human genome ended in a tie. On June 26, 2000, Venter and Francis Collins (then head of the NIH sponsored Human Genome Project) stood next to President Bill Clinton and heard him declare: "today we are here to celebrate the first complete survey of the entire human genome ... with this profound knowledge humankind is on the verge of gaining immense, new power to heal. Genome science ... will revolutionize the diagnosis, prevention and treatment of most, if not all, human diseases."

By 1992, in the UK, the Wellcome Trust was beginning to develop an interest in genome sequencing. In that same year, a chance meeting between David Kemp (then at the Walter and Eliza Hall Institute, WEHI) and Alistair Craig (then at Oxford University) at a Keystone Conference in Utah resulted in the suggestion that there be a coordinated effort by several laboratories engaged in DNA sequencing to sequence the malaria genome. This dovetailed nicely with the subsequent establishment (1994) of the Sanger Centre, dedicated to genome sequencing, within the Wellcome Trust Genome Campus (at Hinxton). Information on the number and size of malaria parasite chromosomes became available only after the development of pulsed-field gel electrophoresis a clever technique that permits separation of very large-sized molecules. Using this novel approach, it was possible to separate the 14 chromosomes of *Plasmodium falciparum*. At a meeting on severe malaria sponsored by the Wellcome Trust, Craig, Kemp, and Chris Newbold (Oxford University), approached the Director of the Trust, Bridget Ogilvie, as to whether the Trust would support sequencing the genome of the malaria parasite, *P. falciparum*. The Trust agreed to fund a multi-center collaboration to map ESTs that included from Australia Alan Cowman and David Kemp, from the U.S. Jeffrey Ravetch (then at Rockefeller University), and from the UK Newbold and Tony Holder (NIMR). In 1995, a Trust-sponsored meeting at the new Sanger Centre discussed establishing a Pathogen Sequencing

Unit, under Bart Barrell. At this meeting priorities for sequencing the bacterium causing tuberculosis and *P. falciparum*, were established and monies for a pilot project to sequence the very smallest chromosome (number 1) of *P. falciparum* were provided. In 1996, Barrell and colleagues at the Sanger Centre demonstrated that it was possible to assemble gene sequences from small clones of chromosome 1. This was a proof of principle that was needed for the feasibility and initiation of large-scale sequencing of the 14 *P. falciparum* chromosomes.

Independently, 'across the pond' Stephen L. Hoffman (b. 1948) a lean, green-eyed, exuberant optimist, entertained similar ideas about sequencing malaria genomes.[79] Hoffman received a BA from the University of Pennsylvania (1970) and an MD from Cornell University Medical College (1975) followed by a residency at UC San Diego. Armed with a Diploma in Tropical Medicine from the London School of Hygiene and Tropical Medicine, he spent nearly five years in Jakarta, Indonesia (NAMRU-2) studying tropical diseases, and was then rotated back to the U.S. where he was based at the Naval Medical Research Institute (NMRI) (later named the Naval Medical Research Center, NMRC). There as the Director of its Malaria Program from 1987–2001, he built a team of over 100 individuals in the U.S. and overseas working on all aspects of malaria but especially vaccine development. Hoffman read Venter's papers on the genomes of *Haemophilus* and *Mycoplasma* musing, "Wouldn't it be interesting to do the same with *P. falciparum*?"

At the NMRC was Sarah L. French (b. 1951). In 1993 French, who had received her Ph.D. from the Scripps Institution of Oceanography in La Jolla, was doing post-doctoral training with Oscar L. Miller, Jr. at the University of Virginia, studying chromosome structure and function. Miller was then approaching retirement and in order to continue the service contract on the electron microscope and her research French submitted, on her own, a grant application to the NIH. This narrowly missed funding, and without support, her work couldn't continue. Unable to wait for another round of grant reviews she applied for various advertised positions that sounded interesting. When she read about an open position in the malaria program at NMRC, she felt it dovetailed with her interests in adaptation, and in July Hoffman hired her. In the spring of 1995, she went to TIGR for a seminar that the UC San Francisco biochemist Bruce

Alberts was giving and to speak with him about shared interests in the interaction between DNA replication and transcription. She also had the chance to speak extensively with Craig Venter about a connected interest concerning genome organization and the orientation of genes relative to the direction of replication. It was during this chance conversation that the possibility and importance of sequencing the malaria genome was discussed. Contact information was then shared with Hoffman. Hoffman called Venter to ask whether TIGR had an interest in sequencing the *P. falciparum* and *P. vivax* genomes. When Venter said yes, Hoffman approached one of the scientists on his staff, Malcolm Gardner, to give him a tutorial on ESTs and genomics, before he went to see Venter. Gardner received his Ph.D. (1985) studying murine retroviruses and oncogenes then moved to the NIMR in Mill Hill, England, where he spent six years studying the *P. falciparum* apicoplast. Doing a great deal of manual sequencing and learning how to use computer programs to collect and analyze sequence data were skills that proved useful in the Malaria Genome Project. In 1995, he moved to Hoffman's group at the NMRC to work on *P. yoelii* DNA vaccines. Daniel Carucci aided Gardner in the sequencing efforts at the NMRC. Carucci who joined Hoffman's team in January 1996 received his Medical Degree from the University of Virginia School of Medicine supported by a scholarship from the U.S. Navy. His military stint exposed him to tropical diseases and thereby began a life-long interest in their cure. In 1991, he was awarded a Masters of Science in Clinical Tropical Medicine and in 1995 a Doctor of Philosophy from the London School of Hygiene & Tropical Medicine. At the NMRC he was responsible for the creation of the Malaria Genomics and Applied Genomics Laboratory, and was the Director of the Malaria Vaccine Program leading the U.S. Navy's efforts in the development and testing of malaria vaccines.

The fond hope of the Malaria Genome Project was that the gene sequence would 'provide a road map for malaria research in the 21st century, research that will lead to improved treatment and prevention', however, at the time there was no common fund to support the sequencing efforts in the U.S. Hoffman went over to TIGR, discussed the project with Venter, and they agreed a concerted effort would have to be made to obtain the $28 million in funding Venter estimated the project would cost.

In late December of 1995 Venter and Hoffman elected to hold a meeting at TIGR's headquarters to 'set the ball in motion' and to delineate the necessary steps to obtain funds, however, it was a meeting that nearly did not come about. The meeting was scheduled for Saturday January 6, 1996. On that day, snow began falling on Washington, DC ushering in the blizzard of 1996. "The entire region was shut down. High winds caused snow to blow back onto plowed roads and many streets were not plowed at all. The Metro system fared no better as frozen rails crippled the outside portion of that system. One train with 100 passengers on board, got stuck for four hours near Takoma Park" (http://www.weatherbook.com/1996. htm) Maryland. "A four car Red Line Metrorail train overran the Shady Grove Station Platform and plowed into an unoccupied six-car train, killing the operator. Thousands of people were without electricity" (http:// washington examiner.com/local/remembering-blizzard-03996). President Clinton shut down the government. Undaunted by the fierce weather the government's Navy men (Hoffman, Gardner and Carucci) and William Bancroft, Head of the Military Infectious Disease Program at Ft. Detrick, MD, trudged through drifts of snow (which in some places had accumulated to two feet) to get to TIGR's headquarters in Maryland. The justification for the involvement of Department of Defense (Navy and Army) was that sequencing would accelerate the development of a protective vaccine (as well as drugs) for malaria!

In March, after giving a 20-minute presentation at the NIH on the Project Hoffman was able to garner a million dollars in funding. TIGR wrote an addendum to its NIH grant on sequencing the genome of tuberculosis and received additional monies for the malaria project. Venter contacted the Burroughs Wellcome Fund and they too promised funds. By May, with interest already expressed in the UK by the Sanger and the Wellcome Trust, an international consortium of scientists and funding agencies was established. The NMRI was to provide DNA and chromosomes, and TIGR, Stanford University and the Sanger would do the sequencing. Coordination of activities would be through e-mails, conference calls and two meetings a year — one in the U.S. (at the ASTMH meeting) and another in the UK. By September in conjunction with the annual meeting of the ASTMH it was announced that $28 million had been committed by the various donor agencies for the Malaria Genome Project.[79]

The Sanger Centre and TIGR were not only competitors — some would describe them as enemies — the two had very different philosophies. In 1993, John Sulston was the Director of the Sanger Centre, and during a visit to the U.S. he met Venter who was focused on sequencing more and faster, and intent on moving into the private sector.[80] Sulston was personally offended by Venter's competitive streak and he regarded the research being done at TIGR as a challenge to what the Sanger Centre was doing. There were other problems. TIGR was set up as a private, non-profit genome center funded by a venture capital group that established Human Genome Sciences Inc. to develop and market products from TIGR discoveries. Venter predicted finding a thousand genes daily. Sulston regarded Venter's approach to be a compromise of his academic integrity and felt Venter wanted it both ways: recognition and acclaim from his scientific peers, but also secrecy to help his business partners and ultimately to enjoy the profits. Sulston's view was that the results of a genome project were to provide as much information as possible that could be used by everyone, public and private, to advance understanding. The real danger, as he saw it, was that if companies selling drugs or diagnostic kits were to gain exclusive rights to genomic sequences it would prevent others down the line from having any incentive to use the information in creative ways thus impoverishing science and medicine. The Wellcome Trust as a charity shared this view. Indeed, its absolute rule was that the sequence data generated at the Sanger Centre would be immediately released into the public domain. The Trust went a step further and categorically stated they were opposed to patenting the basic genome information and would be prepared to contest such in the courts. Despite this, patenting of gene sequences (initially a practice at the NIH but later discarded) would be open to those who made the discovery of a sequence's function and for the development of commercial products. There were deep suspicions among the gene sequencers regarding Venter's motives. Sulston has written caustically: "part of the reason why people find Craig hard to stomach, and why others admire him greatly, is his cavalier disregard for academic niceties." "Craig was in a business and the priority for business is not scientific credibility but share price and market penetration."[80] The Sanger Centre was on its guard for the challenge from TIGR especially since Barrell's team had beaten them in completing the sequence of the tubercle bacillus. However, to some participants — in what has been described as a 'mud-wrestling match' — it wasn't a matter of racing to be the first and claiming glory, there was the looming danger that control of a genome sequence might reside in private hands.[80]

There followed many meetings in an attempt to reconcile the differences between the 'gene hunters' and their respective institutions and in time, several funding agencies came together to finance and help manage the groups that would undertake the sequencing efforts as well as to assist in establishing the policies on data release and access. The result was a policy that balanced the rights and responsibilities of the sequencers to analyze and publish their results with the opportunities that rapid release of the genomic sequence data would provide to other investigators. This policy on data release and access has since become the guideline for other sequencing projects.

Due to the large size of the *P. falciparum* genome and the large cost of the project it was reasoned that the efforts of all the members of the consortium would be needed to sequence all the genes in all 14 chromosomes. In May 1996 at a meeting sponsored by the NIH and the Burroughs Wellcome Fund scientists and potential funders met to discuss the possibility of using a chromosome-by-chromosome shotgun sequencing approach. The result of the meeting was a plan to divide the work by chromosome with about half the work being done in the U.S. and half in the UK. A pilot project at TIGR and the NMRC, funded by NIH and the U.S. Department of Defense, was dedicated to sequencing chromosome 2. Sequencing of chromosome 12 was undertaken at Stanford University with support from the Burroughs Wellcome Fund, and at the Sanger Centre (Cambridge, United Kingdom) Patricia Goodwin from Wellcome acted effectively and collegially with the NIAID on coordinating the effort and a pilot project was launched at the Sanger Centre to sequence chromosome 3. Eventually, the distributed parasite genome sequencing projects were: the Sanger Centre with chromosomes 1, 3–9, and 13, TIGR with chromosomes 2, 10, 11, and 14, and Stanford University with chromosome 12. Early on the sequencers encountered surprisingly difficult problems. Indeed, Malcolm Gardner said the project to sequence the nuclear genome of *P. falciparum* was a 'real nightmare', because of the parasite's unusually high proportion (~89%) of A and T in the coding region of the DNA that made it difficult to clone the genetic material in bacteria and to sequence it. Nevertheless, with the development of new techniques and software the problem of sequencing an AT-rich genome was eventually overcome. Chromosome 2 was the first chromosome fully sequenced and this was published in 1998 by the TIGR–NMRC team.[81] The sequence of chromosome 3 came a year later by the Sanger-Oxford team[82] and the entire *P. falciparum* genome sequence in 2002.[83]

On occasion, the meetings at which members of the sequencing centers, funders and collaborators met to discuss progress and exchange data could be quite tense affairs. A notable one was at the Fourth Malaria Genome Sequencing Meeting, Orlando, Florida December 11–12, 1997, where a heated discussion between the sequencing partners at Oxford University and the NMRC led to some pushing, shoving and chest bumping interactions in which neither party came out looking very well. The 11th Meeting was held at the Sanger Centre in 2001. After the day-long formal discussions, some of the attendees repaired to the local Red Lion pub. After the pub closed, informal discourse continued back at the bar in the main house, with the bartender manning the bar until midnight, when the door to the bar was locked. Not content with the amounts of alcohol that had been consumed during the evening, the remaining sequencing center revelers scaled the top of the bar and grabbed bottles of single malt whiskey to continue the 'discussions' into the wee hours. At the next year's meeting, a metal security gate appeared over the bar!

In 1998, Venter left TIGR and the *P. falciparum* Genome Project to become the President of Celera Genomics, a for profit company dedicated to sequencing the human genome. A year prior to Venter's departure it was decided that it would be optimal to have Gardner move from the NMRC to TIGR to work on the *P. falciparum* genome project full-time. A Brazilian scientist, Leda Cummings joined Gardner and a very talented post-doctoral fellow Herve Tettelin in the sequencing project. Tetellin had received a degree in Industrial Engineer in Biotechnology from the Institut Seperieur Industriel del la Province de Liege, Belgium and a B.S. and Ph.D. in Applied Sciences for the Universite Catholique de Louvain, Belgium.

At TIGR Tettelin became the primary person responsible for the sequence analysis of the *P. falciparum* chromosome 2. Hoffman, was also keen for TIGR to sequence the genome of the rodent malaria model *P. yoelii*, as a means to jump-start gene finding in a rodent model used for immunological studies at NMRC — and at TIGR Cummings took on the role as the principal investigator of this project. However, things did not quite go as planned. The working relationship between Gardner and Cummings was, to say the very least, strained. Indeed, Venter had, on more than one occasion, summoned both of them into his office and demanded they work their issues out, or else. This deteriorating relationship culminated in Cummings leaving TIGR in the Spring of 2001 to join the Computational Biology Branch (CBB) of the National Center for Biotechnology Information (NCBI) at NIH. Ironically, Jane Carlton (b. 1967) was also at CBB but desperate to find a way out and be a part of the malaria genome projects. The two female scientists overlapped at NCBI for three weeks before Carlton left to join TIGR. At the time, it was rumored that the ever-competitive Venter had said, TIGR won the Cummings–Carlton swap; in the process Carlton inherited the project to sequence the genome of *P. yoelii* and also worked on the sequencing of the falciparum and vivax genomes.

Carlton was admirably suited for the task of genome sequencing. Carlton graduated in 1990 with a B.S. in genetics from Edinburgh University. She then joined David Walliker's malaria genetics group at Edinburgh University for her Ph.D. studying the inheritance of particular genes using the rodent malaria *P. chabaudi*. After receiving the Ph.D. (1995) she spent another two years in Edinburgh analyzing genetic crosses for chloroquine and mefloquine resistance. In 1997, Carlton moved to John Dame's laboratory at the University of Florida where it was realized for the first time that ESTs (short ~500 nucleotide tags) would be useful for gene discovery; Carlton and Dame began using ESTs to begin sequencing *P. vivax*, *P. berghei*, as well as *P. falciparum*. After a brief stay at the NCBI she was appointed to the faculty of TIGR where she helped to complete the *P. falciparum* genome sequence.

In 2000, Hoffman was recruited to Celera Genomics to become Vice President of Biologics with the intent of turning the human genome sequences into immunotherapeutics for cancer. While there, and with Venter's support and a $9 million NIH grant, the sequencing of the

Anopheles gambiae genome was begun. Despite the genome of *A. gambiae* being 10 times larger than *P. falciparum* the sequencing was completed in 40 days. On October 2, 2002 just a day before publication of the *Plasmodium* and *Anopheles* genomes, a press meeting was called to announce this land-mark event. This required an intense amount of coordination, since it involved several genome sequencing centers (TIGR, Stanford, Sanger), several funders (Wellcome Trust, Burroughs Wellcome Fund, the U.S. Department of Defense and NIAID/NIH), both *Nature* (publishing the *Plasmodium* genome papers) and *Science* (publishing the *A. gambiae* genome), as well as numerous collaborators.[83,84] The press meetings were held in both the UK and U.S., with representatives from each of the centers flying to both places to provide an equal presence. After the press meetings, the UK celebrations were predictably raucous. The TIGR/NMRC team in contrast had a rather short-lived and staid lunch with the *Science* editors and Berriman of the Sanger Centre. The celebration was completed by mid-afternoon — most likely in time for all concerned to get back to their desks and continue hunting genes.

The press interest in the completion of the malaria and mosquito genome projects was intense, however, it was short lived. On October 3, 2002 a shooting spree in a suburb of Maryland by the Beltway Snipers made the headlines and bumped the malaria genomes off the front page. Gardner ruefully quoted the pop-artist Andy Warhol and said this ended his 15 minutes of fame.

Undoubtedly the success of the *Plasmodium* genome projects was accelerated by the injection of 'new blood' into the project in 2000/2001. In early 2000, in addition to Barrell, the project at Sanger was taken on by Neil Hall, a young, motivated and highly agreeable scientist who made friends easily especially among those he respected. Neil's particular friendship with Director of Bioinformatics Owen White at TIGR (fueled by their mutual interest in a convivial night on the town and good science) helped smooth the interactions between TIGR and Sanger. (Indeed, Hall left Sanger and joined TIGR in 2003, spent two years there, and then returned to the UK). At TIGR, Carlton's camaraderie with her fellow com-patriots at the Sanger facilitated the exchange of ideas and greater collabo-ration. And, Matt Berriman, No. 2 at the Sanger Centre, had spent several years as a parasitology post-doctoral fellow in the U.S. The camaraderie between the two groups was cemented even further during the week after the September 11, 2001 terrorist attack on New York and Washington, DC. Hall and Berriman were stranded in Boston after the meeting they were to attend was canceled. Since airspace was shut down, the TIGR team invited them down to Washington, DC so that their trip would not be in vain. Driving through the back roads between Boston and DC, they made it to TIGR and spent the next few days accepting TIGR hospitality, before flying back to the UK. They were enormously pleased to have been invited and the relationship between the two sequencing centers flourished.

The results of the *P. falciparum* Genome Project postulated 5,279 genes that code for ~5,300 proteins. It was found that about 60% of these proteins lack any similarity to proteins found in other living organisms; these are referred to as hypothetical proteins. The question was: of these proteins, which might serve as a possible protective antigen?

Chapter 8

Developing Vaccines Against Blood Stages

All of the pathology of malaria relates to parasites multiplying and destroying red blood cells. The concept of a blood stage vaccine is based on a fundamental principle: mimic the immunity that occurs in nature. In falciparum-endemic areas natural acquired immunity is induced by continued exposure to the bite of infected anopheline mosquitoes and although malaria parasites persist in the blood, successive bouts of clinical disease are diminished due to reduced parasite reproduction. Proponents of a blood stage vaccine for falciparum malaria assume it will adversely affect parasite multiplication so as to reduce the parasite burden thereby limiting disease severity and death.

i. Duffy Binding Proteins (DBPs)

The molecular mechanisms of entry into the red blood cell have been considered the Achilles heel of the malaria parasite to be exploited for the development of a protective vaccine. However, despite more than a half century of 'invasion research' a practical and effective means for interrupting the entry process into red blood cells is yet to be achieved.

Despite the fact that the invasion of red blood cells by merozoites was described in studies carried out at WRAIR in 1969 it took six more years and technical improvements in electron microscopy to provide a detailed description of the process using *P. knowlesi*. Other electron microscopic studies have shown similar structural characteristics for erythrocytic merozoites including *Plasmodium falciparum* and *P. vivax*. (Figure 1).

At the pointed tip of the *Plasmodium* merozoite and within its cytoplasm is a pair of membrane-bound pear-shaped and ducted structures called rhoptries; more numerous (up to 40) fusiform bodies that converge around the ends of the rhoptry ducts, called micronemes, and spheroidal

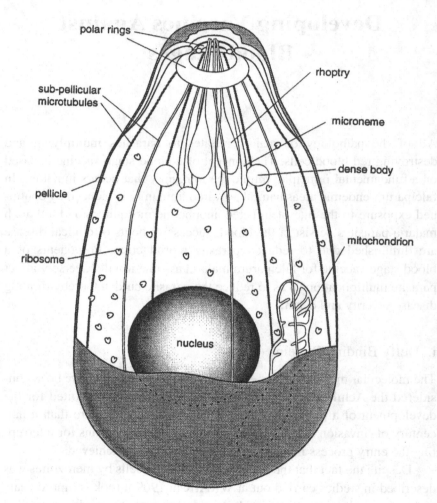

Figure 1.   The merozoite (diagrammatic).

membranous vesicles, the dense granules. The surface of the merozoite is covered with an electron dense fibrillar coat. Primary attachment of the merozoite occurs at any point on the merozoite surface, and then there is re-orientation so that the tip is juxtaposed to the red blood cell surface. At the point of contact with the red cell an electron dense area is seen beneath the red cell membrane. The electron dense area, termed a "tight junction," forms a circumferential ring around the merozoite. (The components and constituents of the junction are not known.) During invasion the rhoptries discharge their contents, the ends of the ducts fuse with each other and the merozoite plasma membrane, and then they collapse. The micronemes also release their contents. Concomitant with rhoptry–microneme discharge the tight junction moves from the front end of the merozoite to the back end powered by its actin–myosin motor and in the process the merozoite's fuzzy coat is shed. As the tight junction moves backwards the molecules mediating invasion (see below) are removed by one or more enzymes. With the discharge of the contents of the rhoptries, the red cell membrane begins to expand allowing the merozoite to induce an invagination; when this is sealed, it forms an enclosing membrane separating the parasite from the red cell cytoplasm. (Think of this as a finger being poked into a semi-inflated balloon — the balloon being the red cell, the finger the merozoite, and the rubber of the balloon around the finger is the membrane.) The entire process of merozoite entry into a red blood cell is quick: it takes less than 30 seconds.

As an NIH post-doctoral fellow at the Rockefeller Institute in New York City one of the projects I undertook was to identify the red blood cell receptor for the merozoites of *P. lophurae*. Prior to my work, Barclay McGhee (then at the Rockefeller Institute in Princeton, NJ) had also tried to find the receptor. The idea was to remove the receptor by various enzyme treatments of the red blood cells and then determine which of these treatments affected merozoite invasion. For example, if the enzyme neuraminidase, which removes sialic acid from the red cell surface, was effective in blocking invasion then it would be reasonable to conclude that sialic acid was a receptor. He introduced duckling red blood cells stripped of their surface molecules into the chick embryo by intravenous inoculation into the chorioallantoic veins of embryos infected with *P. lophurae* and measured the invasion rate of merozoites into the treated red blood cells. None of the enzyme treatments McGhee tried blocked merozoite invasion.[85] However, what McGhee's experiments did show was that the merozoite did not simply bump into any red blood cell and then enter, rather it was quite selective in the particular kind of red cell it would invade — preferring duck over chick red blood cells.

Injecting blood cells into the chorioallantoic veins of a chick embryo requires considerable skill and although I had been a student in Experimental Embryology at Northwestern University this was a technique I had never tried. Instead of embryos, I elected to use an *in vitro* system that Trager had previously employed (as well as one used by a Harvard group in the 1940s). This method uses highly synchronous growing parasites removed from the duckling, placing these in a small Erlenmeyer flask containing various media, and then adding enzyme treated red blood cells. This system avoids host immune reactions and by taking blood samples from the flask, making a blood smear, staining, and then counting the infected red blood cells by light microscopy, a distinction between *in vitro* growth and merozoite invasion is possible. Once the flasks were assembled with medium and enzyme-treated cells they were placed on a rocking table to keep the red blood cells in suspension, placed in an incubator at 38–40°C and each flask received a gas mixture: 95% air and 5% CO_2. Using such *in vitro* cultures I found it impossible to block the invasion of *lophurae* merozoites into duckling red cells by pre-treatment with enzymes in order to strip them of their putative merozoite receptors.[86] This failure was, I believe, due to the agitation of the red blood cells which was detrimental to merozoite invasion, the medium and gas mixture were wrong, but most importantly there was a very high affinity of the lophurae merozoites for the duckling red blood cell. I had chosen the wrong model system!

Although I abandoned further work on red blood cell receptors for merozoite invasion others did not. One of these was Louis H. Miller. Miller (b. 1935) received a B.S. degree from Haverford College (Pennsylvania) in 1956 and an M.D. from Washington University (St. Louis) in 1960. Miller's interest in tropical medicine was piqued by reading the autobiography, "Out of My Life and Thoughts," by Nobelist Albert Schweitzer. After an internship and residency in internal medicine at the Mt. Sinai Medical Center in New York (1960–1964) he spent a year at Cedars-Sinai Medical Center in Los Angeles as a renal metabolism fellow, training that would stand him in good stead for later studies on renal pathology in human and experimental malarias. Returning to New York City he worked with Harold Brown (Head of Parasitology and Tropical Medicine at Columbia University School of Public Health who had spent most of his life working in tropical medicine.) receiving a Master's degree in Parasitology in 1965. Drafted into the U.S. Army as a Captain in the Medical Corps he was sent to WRAIR's SEATO Laboratory in Bangkok, Thailand where he intended to study tropical sprue, however, after encountering only a single case in two years he felt it wise to seek other pathologies. At that time chloroquine-resistant malaria was a significant problem for the troops fighting in Vietnam and so Miller, the clinician, turned his attention from tropical sprue to malaria. Knowing little about malaria he spent a month in the library in Bangkok learning all he could. Comparative studies on the pathology and renal physiology using monkeys and rodents as well as deep vascular schizogony and sequestration were carried out with Robert Desowitz (who had been a student of the malariologist Colonel Henry E. Shortt at the London School and later was on the faculty at the University of Hawaii). After completion of military service Miller joined the faculty at the Columbia University. In 1971 Miller left Columbia University to establish a malaria lab at the NIH.

Shortly after joining the NIH Miller attended a conference organized by Elvio Sadun at WRAIR and there he met Sydney Cohen (from Guy's Hospital in London) who was carrying out short-term cultures of *P. knowlesi* to study invasion In 1973, Geof Butcher, Sydney Cohen, and Graham Mitchell (with support from the Medical Research Council (MRC) and World Health Organization (WHO)), used an *in vitro* short-term culture system to study merozoite invasion and found that red cells from Old World monkeys (kra and rhesus) were susceptible to *P. knowlesi* merozoites whereas New World monkey (*Aotus*) and human red cells were less susceptible and non-primates were completely resistant.[87] This suggested to Miller that it might be possible to use enzymatic treatment of red blood cells (a la McGhee and Sherman) to define the chemical nature of a red blood cell membrane receptor. When human red cells were treated with chymotrypsin or pronase invasion of *P. knowlesi* merozoites was blocked whereas neuraminidase and trypsin were ineffective.[88] However, rhesus red cells treated with the chymotrypsin remained susceptible. Miller *et al.* suggested the differences in invasion between the two kinds of red cells were due to the "high affinity between *P. knowlesi* merozoites and (rhesus) monkey erythrocytes (which) may require greater alteration of the receptor to inhibit invasion."[89] The study allowed for the formulation of a hypothesis: by identification of the red cell receptor it might be possible to isolate the merozoite component that initiates invasion, and once isolated susceptible individuals could be immunized to prevent merozoite penetration into the red blood cell.

Miller and coworkers took advantage of the availability of human red cells that differed genetically in their surface molecules (something lacking for duckling erythrocytes) and was able to show that *P. knowlesi* merozoites could invade human red cells that have the Duffy factor antigen (called Duffy positive) on their surface, but if human red cells lacked the Duffy antigen they were refractory.[88] Then, using enzyme "stripping"[89] it was found that when Duffy antigen was removed from human red cells by chymotrypsin (but not trypsin or neuraminidase) treatment the erythrocytes became Duffy negative and these cells resisted invasion by *P. knowlesi* merozoites.

A visit to the library led Miller to hypothesize that the factor for the resistance of West Africans to *P. vivax* must be a preponderance of Duffy negativity. The basis for this is: (1) West Africans and black Africans who are 95% and 70% Duffy negative respectively were resistant to *P. vivax*, (2) Duffy negative volunteers failed to become infected when bitten by mosquitoes carrying *P. vivax*, and (3) Of 13 black Americans who had vivax malaria in Vietnam all were found to be Duffy positive.[90] (Final and direct proof of Miller's hypothesis came when a short-term culture of *P. vivax* showed the merozoites did not invade Duffy negative cells.)[91]

Human Duffy antigen (similar to the Rh antigen and the A and B blood group antigens) is a protein with two sugar molecules and the sugars are removed when the red blood cells are treated with the enzyme neuraminidase. However, under natural conditions Duffy negativity is not due to an absence of the sugars but results from a gene mutation (cytosine to thymine) on the Duffy gene that does away with the binding site for a transcription factor and as a result transcription of Duffy mRNA in red blood cells but no other cell types is abolished.[92] Although the Duffy determinant has been shown to be crucial for the entry of vivax merozoites recent observations indicate that this pathway is not absolute i.e. *P. vivax* infections were found in two Duffy negative individuals from South America[93] and in four Duffy negative individuals from East Africa.[94] This suggests that *P. vivax* merozoites are able (albeit infrequently) to infect Duffy negative red cells and in this species, as in *P. falciparum*, alternate pathways for invasion of the red cell do exist.

Chetan Chitnis (b. 1961) did undergraduate work in Physics at the Indian Institute of Technology (IIT), Bombay, a Master's in Physics at Rice University (1985), and a Ph.D. from UC Berkeley (1990) working on the biosynthetic pathway of the polysaccharide alginate, an important virulence factor, in *Pseudomona aeruginosa*. He joined Miller's NIH laboratory for post-doctoral work in 1991. When he arrived at the NIH the merozoite genes encoding the DBP for *P. vivax* and *P. knowlesi* (PvDBP and PkDBP) had been identified by John Adams. Moreover, Adams had demonstrated by sequence analysis that all these genes belonged to a family of erythrocyte binding proteins (EBPs), named the DBPs. The *P. vivax* DBP is a 140,000 dalton (140 kDa) protein located in the apical organelles of the merozoite called micronemes. Miller gave Chetan the task of identifying the receptor-binding domains of the *P. vivax* DBP. To do this Chitnis developed an assay in which the various domains (I–V) could be expressed on the surface of a fibroblast derived from an African green monkey kidney cell line (COS cells). The COS cells expressing a 330-amino acid cysteine-rich domain referred to as region II of PvDBP bound Duffy positive human red cells with specificity.[95,96] Chetan returned to India in 1995 to start his own lab at the International Center for Genetic Engineering and Biotechnology (New Delhi) where he continues to work on these binding proteins, to understand their functional roles as well as to explore the possibility of developing vaccines based on these proteins. His recent work focuses on the *P. falciparum* reticulocyte binding-like homolog protein (PfRH5) a promising vaccine candidate (see p. 142).

Because anti-PvDBP antibodies are found in individuals living in malaria-endemic areas, that their concentration increases with the age of the individual, and boosting occurs with repeated exposure to infected mosquitoes it supports the view that DBP might induce a protective immune response during *P. vivax* infections.[97,98]

Large amounts of PvDBP (PvRII) can be produced in the laboratory and rabbit antibodies raised against a recombinant protein are able to inhibit merozoite invasion of human red blood cells it was suggested that PvRII might serve as a possible vaccine candidate for *P. vivax*. Indeed, it has been demonstrated that naturally acquired antibodies elicited against PvDBP did block the binding of PvRII to Duffy positive human red cells although the binding inhibitory activity was poor.[98,99] High titer antibodies against PvRII do not develop upon natural exposure to *P. vivax*, but it is possible to raise high titer antibodies by immunization with recombinant PvRII; partial protection of *Aotus* monkeys against *P. vivax* has also been achieved when PvRII was formulated with Freund's complete antigen (FCA). Other adjuvant formulations with PvRII (Montanide ISA720 and ASO2 and allohydrogel) were found to be safe and immunogenic in Rhesus monkeys and all had significant binding inhibitory activity.[100] Although PvDBP is a relatively poor imunogen and strain-transcending immunity is uncommon (because of DBP polymorphism) it is possible to produce a highly immunogenic and specific binding synthetic antigen lacking all the polymorphic residues. This suggests that such an antigen might be able to avoid strain-specific immune responses[101,102] and could serve as a putative protective vaccine.

ii. Erythrocyte Binding Antigen 175 (EBA-175)

By the early 1980s — a time when *P. falciparum* could be cultured continuously in the laboratory — there was mounting evidence that the receptor for *P. falciparum* differed from that of *P. vivax* and *P. knowlesi*.[103] Several laboratories reported that a red blood cell receptor for *P. falciparum* merozoites was sialic acid (N-acetylneuraminic acid) since human red blood cells treated with neuraminidase or trypsin resisted invasion by *P. falciparum* merozoites and this was unlike the situation with *P. vivax* and *P. knowlesi* where "stripping" by chymotrypsin but not trypsin blocked invasion (see above). Further, Tn red blood cells which lack a glycosyltransferase that results in red cells deficient in sialic acid were also refractory to invasion, as were En (a–) cells; and when and S–s– U (–) red cells which were relatively resistant to invasion were treated with trypsin they became totally resistant.[104] These studies suggested (but did not prove) that glycophorin A, a sialic-acid bearing glycoprotein, was the red blood cell receptor for *P. falciparum* merozoites.

The physician, Terence Hadley (b. 1941), after finishing a medical internship and residency at the University of Florida practiced general medicine in Africa (Nigeria) where he came in contact with many cases of malaria, especially in young children some of whom arrived at the clinic suffering with seizures. This piqued an interest in malaria research and upon return to the U.S., and after reading Louis Miller's papers on the Duffy antigen and *P. vivax*, Hadley decided to join Miller's NIH laboratory. There he worked on the characterization of the Duffy antigen. Later, when he moved from Miller's lab to WRAIR (and had to join the U.S. Army!) the military wanted Hadley to focus on *P. falciparum*. At WRAIR he met with a Senior Research Associate of the National Research Council, the Frenchman, Daniel Camus, who was studying (for diagnostic purposes) the malaria antigens found in the supernatants of *P. falciparum* cultures. It was known at the time (1985) that glycophorin was a receptor for invasion by *P. falciparum*, however other laboratories were unable to identify the merozoite ligand using purified glycophorin as an affinity substrate. Perhaps, they mused, the merozoite ligand might be shed into the culture supernatant and would bind to intact red blood cells where the glycophorin receptor would be in the correct native conformation. They designed an experiment: radioactive isoleucine (an essential amino acid for *P. falciparum*) was added for four hours to schizont-infected red blood cells from synchronized cultures of *P. falciparum* in order to label the merozoite proteins; the supernatants from the culture were collected, and incubated with a variety of intact uninfected red blood cells as well as enzyme treated red blood cells; then the red cells were washed, lysed, and precipitated with serum from a Nigerian donor containing malaria antibodies. The various immunoprecipitated proteins (antigens) bearing radioactivity were separated by electrophoresis and visualized on X-ray film. Of the four antigens recovered only one, at a molecular size of 175,000 Daltons (175 kDa), bound to intact normal human red blood cells but not to neuraminidase treated red blood cells, nor Ena (1-) nor Tn cells and it specifically bound to glycophorin. Because of its molecular size and its red blood cell (=erythrocyte) binding the antigen was named EBA-175. On the basis of the specific binding Hadley and Camus postulated that the

175 kDa antigen could be involved in the initial step of recognition by the merozoite and in a prescient fashion wrote "understanding the molecules involved in invasion may contribute to the development of a malaria vaccine."[105]

EBA-175 is a micronemal protein encoded by a single copy gene located on chromosome 7. EBA-175 is divided into six regions (RI–RV) and a cytoplasmic tail. It is the RII region that is critical to binding to the sialic acid on glycophorin A. Targeted disruption (a so-called 'knockout') of the EBA-175 gene in the falciparum clone W2mef whose invasion is sialic acid dependent was associated with a switch to a sialic acid independent pathway of invasion. However, when EBA-175 was disrupted in another cloned line (Dd2/Nm) selected on neuraminidase treated red cells the knockouts invaded the treated cells, as did the wild type.[106] Such findings suggest that *P. falciparum* can invade red blood cells without the involvement of EBA-175 except in one parasite clone. In field isolates from The Gambia and Brazil the sialic acid-dependent pathway of merozoite invasion seems to predominate whereas in India and Kenya neuraminidase and trypsin sensitive, chymotrypsin-resistant receptors (characteristic of EBA-175 mediated invasion) were rarely used.[107]

Naturally acquired antibodies against EBA-175 are found in individuals resident in areas where malaria is endemic and these antibodies protect against symptomatic malaria.[108–110] When antibodies against conserved regions III–V of EBA-175 were produced in rabbits the sera blocked merozoite invasion *in vitro*.[111] In 2010 a trial of the safety and immunogenicity of a recombinant EBA-175 vaccine with alum adjuvant was tested in healthy young adults living in the United States. Eighteen subjects/group received ascending doses (5, 20, 80, or 160 μg) of the vaccine at 0, 1, and 6 months; eight subjects received placebo. Most of the reactions at the injection site (as well as systemic reactions) were mild to moderate in intensity. After two or three doses of the vaccine at any concentration, antibody levels measured by enzyme-linked immunosorbent assay were significantly higher than those for the placebo group. Sera from subjects who received three doses of the vaccine at any concentration inhibited the *in vitro* growth of asexual-stage *P. falciparum* at low levels when compared to sera from placebo recipients or preimmune sera.[112] Thus, the EBA-175 vaccine with adjuvant was safe and immunogenic in malaria-naive subjects.

Because of the technical difficulties associated with expressing full-length *Plasmodium* recombinant proteins in a functionally active and soluble form much of the work on EBA-175 has used just the RII fragment. A recent study reports that it is possible to express the full-length ectodomain of EBA-175 in a soluble recombinant form that is biochemically active and has binding properties similar to the native EBA-175. Antibodies raised against the full-length protein were able to inhibit parasite invasion more potently than antibody raised against the RII fragment, suggesting it might be a better vaccine candidate than the intact RII.[113] To date no clinical evaluation of this has been made.

iii. Monoclonal Antibodies and Merozoite Surface Protein (MSP)-1

a. Discovery of Monoclonal Antibodies

In the 1950s it had become evident that a particular kind of white blood cell, a B lymphocyte, played a key role in the antibody response to a pathogen. There are millions of B cells in our body and each has the capacity to make a particular antibody that is able to recognize a different antigenic determinant (epitope). It is this capacity of lymphocytes to react to each component of a pathogen that is the basis of immune protection. Under ordinary circumstances it is impossible to use immune serum to isolate a particular antigen because it contains a mixture of antibodies directed against a spectrum of antigens. However, were it possible to isolate a particular B lymphocyte from the others, place this in a test tube containing a nutrient medium allowing growth and division into identical progeny (clone) and secreting antibody against a single epitope there would be a "molecular tweezer" able to pluck out a specific antigen. Although theoretically it might be possible to locate and isolate an individual B cell using a microscope and pipette and then place this in culture it would not serve to provide antibody in reasonable amounts because a B cell divides for a finite length of time, the progeny secrete antibody, and then they die. Therefore, to provide abundant amounts of an antigen-selecting antibody required something unnatural — long-lived and dividing lymphocytes that continued to secrete antibody. In 1975 Cesar

Milstein (1926–2002) and Georges Kohler (1927–1995) were able to create this unnatural B lymphocyte.[58]

Milstein, born in a provincial town in Argentina, studied chemistry at the University of Buenos Aires, where he wrote his first Ph.D. thesis on the active site of enzymes. In 1958 he received an MRC scholarship to work in the MRC laboratory of Molecular Biology Cambridge headed by Fred Sanger. Given a small windowless, basement storeroom as his laboratory he turned from enzymes to trying to understand how lymphocytes were able to produce millions of different antibodies. Milstein believed he could solve the problem of antibody diversity by determining the amino acid composition of antibodies and began by using transformed B cells (myelomas) to obtain the amounts necessary for chemical characterization. Myelomas are malignant tumor cells of the immune system that can be grown indefinitely in a test tube and hence are considered "immortal." Although the myelomas in culture produced large amounts of antibody the problem presented to Milstein was that the antibodies made were without specificity.

Kohler, a young, independent Ph.D. student at the Basel Institute of Immunology had been struggling without success to find a way to obtain enough antibodies from mortal B-lymphocytes in culture. After hearing a lecture by Milstein he was convinced that if B lymphocytes making antibody against a known antigen were fused with Milstein's immortalized myeloma cell it would result in a hybrid cell (hybridoma) that could grow indefinitely in culture and secrete antibodies specific for that antigen — designer antibodies. The hybridoma could be maintained indefinitely in the laboratory producing a large amount of identical antibody, called a monoclonal antibody, specific for a single antigenic determinant (epitope). In 1973, Kohler joined the Milstein lab as a post-doctoral fellow and it was shortly thereafter that success was achieved. Once the right components were known the procedure is absurdly simple. Mouse myeloma cells are mixed with spleen cells from a mouse immunized with a particular antigen in the presence of a fusion agent, polyethylene glycol. The desired hybridomas are then selected using a special growth medium and these can be frozen for long-term storage. When a monoclonal antibody is needed the hybridoma is thawed out and injected into mice that provided the original cells for fusion. The mice develop tumors that secrete the specific monoclonal antibody and the serum of such mice also contains a high concentration of antibody (>10 mg/ml serum).

In 1975, Kohler and Milstein submitted their work for publication and although the referee reports were positive the editors of *Nature* did not consider it of sufficient general interest to publish it as a full article and so the original text was severely pruned to fit the length of a letter. The final sentence in their three-page paper is prescient for understatement: "such cultures could be valuable for medical and industrial use." However, the scientific community at large paid little notice. By the time Kolhler and Milstein received the 1984 Nobel Prize for Physiology or Medicine "for the discovery of the production of monoclonal antibodies" Kohler had returned to Germany where he held a position at the Max Planck Institute in Freiburg until his sudden death in 1995 and Milstein continued at the MRC Lab in Cambridge until his death in 2002 from an inherited vascular disorder.

In the British tradition Milstein and Kohler did not patent their invention. At the time of their discovery neither employees of nor the MRC itself was allowed to register patents so they sent the unpublished paper to a patent officer of the National Research and Development Corporation (NRDC) to consider its patenting potential. The NRDC expressed the view that the work as published was not patentable. Since to develop the invention to a state when it would have been adequately protected further work would have had to be carried out under conditions of secrecy Milstein considered himself extremely lucky he was never asked to work in secrecy or to refrain from sending the myeloma partner (which had actually been obtained from Michael Potter of the NIH) to colleagues over the world. Others, however, did not share their sacrifice of personal gain, and some took out patents.

In addition to their therapeutic advantage (due to high specificity with which they bind to their target antigen with limited side effects) a principal value of hybridoma technology has been the ability to derive an antibody to a single component of a crude mixture of antigens; this opens up the way to purify a single antigen and makes possible a dissection of a mixture of completely unknown substances into its components. When wed to molecular biology and recombinant DNA monoclonal antibodies have also been of particular significance to discover and purify those malaria parasite antigens that might serve as the basis of a protective vaccine.

b. The Path to MSP-1

In 1977, the recently appointed head of the Division of Immunobiology at the Wellcome Foundation, the immunologist James Howard, was intent to re-build and re-orient the Department of Immunochemistry to better reflect emerging molecular approaches to microbiology and parasitology. George A. M. Cross (b. 1942) received his undergraduate degree in 1964 and his Ph.D. in biochemistry in 1968 from the University of Cambridge, UK, where he held a MRC Research Training Scholarship; he was an Imperial Chemical Industries Fellow during his post-doctoral years and from 1970 to 1977 he worked in the MRC Biochemical Parasitology Unit in Cambridge. Cross first met Howard at a meeting of the Royal Society of Tropical Hygiene and Medicine early in 1977, and after successive meetings, was offered a job at Wellcome to build a group that would include a prominent commitment to malaria immunology/vaccinology. Although he had no formal training with malaria he had a free hand to learn 'on the job.' Cross began by hiring smart experienced and keen young scientists to spearhead malaria research. The first hire was a talented young immunologist, Robert (Robbie) Freeman, who had recently finished his Ph.D. on the immunology of the rodent malaria *P. yoelii*, in Ian Clark's laboratory at the Australian National University in Canberra. Freeman arrived in 1978 and persuaded Cross that *P. yoelii* was a suitable model for human malaria — existing as it did in virulent and less virulent clones — and was capable of being scaled up for biochemical studies. With an excellent supporting staff, especially Avril Trejdosiewicz, who had been hired to run the monoclonal facility, the first monoclonal antibodies to the asexual blood stages of rodent and human malaria parasites were made.

One of Freeman's first contributions was to show that the best way to identify useful and relevant monoclonal antibodies was to screen, from the beginning, by the time-consuming but more informative approach of immunofluorescence microscopy. The next step was to see if any of the monoclonals would suppress a mouse malaria infection. The first experiment involved two monoclonals: one that clearly reacted with the merozoite surface, which might be recognizing a protective antigen, and the other, which recognized a merozoite-internal structure, and was unlikely to be protective. In fact, both monoclonals were strongly protective in 'passive immunization' experiments.[114] The Immunochemistry group then moved rapidly to purify the target antigen by affinity purification, for which the monoclonal worked well. It was at this point that Cross persuaded Anthony Holder, to get involved with the malaria project and contribute his skills in protein purification and analysis.

Anthony Holder (b. 1951) completed undergraduate studies in Biological Sciences, graduating in Biochemistry at the University of East Anglia in Norwich (1972). Subsequently, for his Ph.D. studies (1972–1975) he worked with John Fincham, a well-known geneticist at the University of Leeds, using protein sequencing methodologies to obtain amino acid sequences of NADP-dependent glutamate dehydrogenase from the wild type and various *am* mutants and revertants of *Neurospora crassa*. At that time DNA sequencing was not routinely available and the dansyl-Edman procedure for peptide sequencing was very slow and extremely laborious; several person-years were devoted to obtaining the 452-amino acid sequence of this protein. Wellcome Trust and Royal Society Fellowships allowed a very enjoyable post-doctoral (1975–1978) at the newly rebuilt Carlsberg Laboratory in Copenhagen with studies on the evening primrose, barley and potato–tomato hybrids, as well as generous contributions from the brewery in the form of their products! However, after three years a new job was needed and a serendipitous flick through the back pages of *Nature* revealed a job to work on African trypanosomes with George Cross who had recently moved to the Wellcome Research Laboratories, a pharmaceutical company whose research facilities in South London were often referred to as the 'University of Beckenham.' In this newly founded Molecular Parasitology group the variant surface glycoprotein (VSG) was the molecule of choice and molecular biology was starting to have its pervasive influence. At the same time (1978), Robbie Freeman had joined the group with the specific remit to establish malaria research, particularly using rodent models and developing monoclonal antibodies to define parasite proteins. This led to a productive five-year collaboration and Holder's conversion to malaria research that has continued ever since. A year after Holder joined the Wellcome group, monoclonal antibodies were used to identify a *P. yoelii* merozoite-specific protein with a molecular mass of 235,000.[115] The protein could be purified and prepared in large amounts by using an affinity column: the monoclonal antibody was bound to a column of Sepharose beads, a merozoite extract was poured over the column, and the protein that bound to the column had the same molecular mass. After immunization with this protein in FCA, the mice survived challenge whereas controls died. It was the first time that this had been done and established the principle of a subunit vaccine against malaria. But, Holder and Freeman wondered, was this of any relevance to *P. falciparum*? They answered their own question upon finding a cross-reaction between the *P. yoelii* antigen and a merozoite antigen from *P. falciparum,* and suggested "this 195,000 mol wt *P. falciparum* protein, and its form on the merozoite surface, are ... of considerable interest for malaria vaccine development."[116] They had discovered the first and most abundant MSP, named MSP-1. (MSP-1 has also been called at various times PMMSA, precursor to major merozoite surface antigens, and Pf 195, a *P. falciparum* 195,000 molecular weight antigen, and FMP1, falciparum merozoite protein 1.)

Cross left Wellcome for his present position as a Professor at The Rockefeller University in 1982 (currently he is Emeritus), but was retained as a consultant from 1982–1987, and Robbie Freeman left Wellcome in 1985, to pursue a different career and lifestyle, and died tragically by his own hand eight years later. In 1988, Holder moved to head the Division of Parasitology at the NIMR, however the Wellcome malaria program continued until 1990, when the program was terminated because Wellcome had moved from being owned entirely by a charitable foundation to being partly a public company.

The initial studies on MSP-1 were rapidly expanded to other *Plasmodium spp.* including sequencing of the gene in *P. falciparum.*[117] How could they be sure it was the right gene? Interestingly it was a protein sequence from a fragment of MSP-1 released into culture supernatants that provided the definitive proof. Studies on the processing of MSP-1 followed, particularly with M. J. (Mike) Blackman, and the discovery that a monoclonal antibody isolated by Jana McBride at Edinburgh University directed against one end of the molecule inhibited merozoite invasion of red blood cells, focused attention on this part of the molecule. Human studies, with Eleanor Riley in The Gambia and Roseangela Nwuba in Nigeria, supported the view that this part of the molecule was important as a target of protective immunity and a possible vaccine candidate. With

Irene Ling and Sola Ogun, in parallel to work being carried out by Carole Long, a recombinant ~100 amino acid fragment (MSP-1$_{19}$) of *P. yoelii* MSP-1 was shown to be effective in protecting mice against a parasite challenge infection.

Carole Long (b. 1944) grew up in Syracuse, NY and received her B.S. degree from Cornell University (1965). Given her background — she worked on basic immunochemistry studying antibody affinity and valence while a graduate student at the University of Pennsylvania (Penn) under the direction of Fred Karush, a physical chemist who had moved into antibody structure and function in immunology — it seemed unlikely that she would work on malaria. Indeed, after receiving her Ph.D. (1970), she did post-doctoral training also at Penn in T cell immunology — studies having little to do with malaria. However, as a young Assistant Professor at Hahnemann University School of Medicine (now Drexel University) she met up with William Weidanz, a Professor in the Department of Microbiology and Immunology, who had worked on mouse and bird malarias using various immunodeficiency models to dissect the roles of antibodies and lymphoid cells in protective immune responses against malaria infection. Weidanz asked for some assistance with some immunochemical techniques that were running in Long's laboratory. Soon Long and Weidanz were carrying out analyses of parasite proteins to identify the numerous red blood cell stage targets of antibodies produced by mice that were protected against a challenge infection.

Prompted by the observation that sera from mice immunized by infection could passively protect naive mice against a virulent challenge infection they started producing monoclonal antibodies from the spleens of mice protected by repeated infection. At the time, other laboratories were taking a similar approach, notably that of Anthony Holder at the NIMR. Will Majarian in the Long laboratory was fortunate enough to find one monoclonal antibody that provided significant although partial protective activity when administered to naive mice even after infection with an ordinarily lethal *P. yoelii*. This observation led to a major effort to identify the antigen that was the target of this protective monoclonal antibody. Accomplishing this required the addition of new molecular biological techniques to the laboratory, which was provided by Jim Burns and Akhil Vaidya. After learning to construct and screen phage libraries of parasite DNA, Long and coworkers eventually identified the target of the monoclonal antibody as the major MSP, MSP-1, particularly MSP-1$_{19}$. Long was now in competition with Holder's laboratory which was also focused on this protein.

The challenge for Long remained to produce a recombinant protein that mimicked this portion of MSP-1. At that time (1992) there was little experience with expression of correctly folded recombinant proteins. Initially, producing MSP-1$_{19}$ of *P. yoelii* directly in *E. coli* was unsuccessful, however, eventually a method was worked out for making it as a fusion protein with glutathione-S-transferase (GST) that appeared to be correctly folded. And when Tom Daly in Long's laboratory came to her with the immunization-challenge data that indicated the mice had been partially protected against an otherwise lethal infection, tears came to her eyes because this was the first time that active protection to blood stage malaria infection was elicited by a recombinant protein. Shortly thereafter, a small workshop was held at the NIH to discuss the status of research on MSP-1. When Holder presented his data on MSP-1 it was clear that he was pursuing the same approach as that of Long, however, his laboratory was not as far along with the immunizations. Patrick Farley, a student from Long's laboratory, also an attendee, looked at her after Holder's presentation, and when their preliminary results were presented after him, the tension in the room was palpable. Long's results with MSP-1 were expanded over the years using various rodent models, and others at the NIH and elsewhere attempted to extend them to non-human primates infected with *P. falciparum*. Subsequently her studies moved to production of an MSP-1 protein suitable for human clinical trials, and a number of laboratories continue to work on MSP-1 as a blood-stage vaccine candidate in human malarias.

In 1999 Long moved to NIH to participate in the new efforts there to actually produce and test malaria vaccine candidates in humans. The efforts at the NIH, sparked by NIH Director Harold Varmus and National Institute of Allergy and Infectious Diseases (NIAID) Chief Anthony Fauci, sought to fill that gap between vaccine candidates discovered in the laboratory into process development and clinical testing. In contrast to the situation with HIV, there appeared to be reasons for optimism with a malaria vaccine given the resistance seen in those living in endemic areas and the success in protecting laboratory animals by immunization.

However, making the transition from a University academic laboratory to a quasi-biotechnology system was not easy. A whole new vocabulary had to be learned and then laboratory procedures had to be modified so that the data would suitable for submission to the U.S. Food and Drug Administration as part of Investigational New Drug applications. The learning curve was very steep to transform one's laboratory procedures and to surmount the massive record keeping and paperwork involved.

Long says "Perhaps we were somewhat naive in thinking that a vaccine using a single recombinant protein directed to such sophisticated and complex organisms would elicit protective responses. In the case of the blood stage infections, it is likely that we will have to elicit a complex combination of immune responses to achieve significant protection in children by vaccination. While most existing vaccines are directed to production of specific antibody, the remaining vaccine development challenges such as malaria or tuberculosis or HIV will likely also require cellular responses as well." While by no means the possibilities of recombinant proteins representing blood stage antigens has been exhausted, Long has taken the approach of stepping back to put vaccination efforts in the context of what happens to those who live in malaria endemic areas, asking: what can be learned about the process by which infants and children develop resistance to malaria? A deeper understanding of the relevant immune mechanisms that evolve with time in children and young adults, coupled with elucidation of the strategies that the parasite employs to manipulate the host immune system may illuminate new directions for vaccines for malaria.

During her professional life Carole Long (as well as I) has been witness to some of the best and the worst in human behavior. She has also met interesting people from around the world, been to villages in Africa that have been little affected by time, and privileged to participate in an important global quest. Currently Chief, Malaria Immunology Section, at NIAID Long continues to work on innate and adaptive immune responses using rodent and human malarias, is evaluating CD4 T cell responses to specific malaria antigens in mice and humans and is currently involved in developing a PfRH5-based vaccine with potential to achieve strain transcending efficacy in humans (see p. 142).

MSP-1 is encoded by a single gene on chromosome 9 in *P. falciparum* and is synthesized late in the blood-stage developmental cycle. It has not been possible to "knockout" the gene for MSP-1, suggesting that it is essential for invasion and parasite survival. Sequence analysis shows that MSP-1 contains conserved regions interspersed with polymorphic regions. MSP-1 undergoes extensive proteolytic processing during merozoite formation and soon after merozoite release four fragments, remain as a complex on the merozoite surface with the 42,000 molecular mass protein (MSP-1$_{42}$) being attached via a GPI anchor. A final processing step mediated during invasion cleaves this fragment into 33,000 and 19,000 fragments (=MSP1$_{19}$); the larger fragment is shed from the merozoite surface along with the remainder of the MSP-1 complex whereas the smaller MSP$_{19}$ remains on the merozoite surface during invasion.

Full length MSP-1 has been suggested to bind to red cells in a sialic acid dependent manner, or it may form a complex that binds to band 3 protein (see p. 166). Antibodies directed against MSP-1$_{19}$ block invasion and prevent processing of MSP-1.[118] Since immunization of *Aotus* with recombinant MSP-1$_{42}$ in the presence of FCA partially protected the monkeys against challenge, and appeared to be as effective as whole merozoites, it was suggested to be a blood stage vaccine candidate. Antibodies directed against MSP-1$_{19}$ in mice and monkeys elicited protection against challenge and similar results were reported with antibodies raised against MSP-1$_{42}$.[119] Immunization of *Aotus* monkeys with a recombinant protein MSP-1$_{42}$ produced in *E. coli* resulted in high-titer antibodies and led to protection against an ordinarily lethal challenge with *P. falciparum*. However, with recombinant MSP-1$_{42}$ and MSP-1$_{19}$, protection of *Aotus* was seen only when high antibody titers were obtained using formulations with FCA; indeed only one of seven monkeys required treatment for uncontrolled blood infections.[120]

So what were the results of a 2010 Phase 1 (safety) vaccination trial in adult human volunteers in Kenya using MSP-1$_{42}$ (also called FMP1) in combination with ASO2A (an oil in water emulsion containing 3-deacylated monophosphoryl lipid A and QS21, a saponin-like adjuvant) or Imovax rabies vaccine? Slightly more recipients of the three intramuscular vaccinations at 0, 1, and 2 months of FMP1/AS02A experienced more pain than with the Imovax group but otherwise the two groups were equal.

The Kenyan volunteers already had high pre-existing antibody titers to FMP-1 and the titers increased after each immunizing dose.[121] The vaccine appeared to be well tolerated and immunogenic, but because its efficacy in adults and in children was disappointing further work was abandoned.

A variety of other MSP-1 vaccines have been tested. In 2013 it was reported that two Phase 1 clinical studies were conducted to examine the safety, reactogenicity, and immunogenicity of the FVO allele of MSP-1$_{42}$ in the GSK proprietary adjuvant system AS01 administered intramuscularly at 0, 1, and 2 months: one in the U.S. and, after evaluation of safety data results, one in Western Kenya. The U.S. study was an open-label, dose escalation study of 10 and 50 μg doses of MSP-1$_{42}$ in 26 adults, while the Kenya study, evaluating 30 volunteers, was a double-blind, randomized study of only the 50 μg dose with a rabies vaccine comparator. It was demonstrated that the vaccine was safe and immunogenic in malaria-naive and malaria-experienced populations. High titres of anti-MSP-1 antibodies were induced in both study populations, although a limited number of volunteers whose serum demonstrated significant inhibition of blood-stage parasites as measured by growth inhibition assay was found. In U.S. volunteers, the antibodies generated exhibited better cross-reactivity to heterologous MSP-1 alleles than an MSP1-based vaccine (3D7 allele) previously tested at both study sites.[122] Pre-clinical work on MSP-1 continues to be undertaken.

iv. AMA-1

The demonstration that antibody from rhesus monkeys immune to *P. knowlesi* inhibited the multiplication of the parasites *in vitro* and that passive transfer of immune monkey serum also conferred protection provided a rationale for using sera from immune hosts to characterize antigens and identify those with putative protective activity.[57] Since it had already been shown that vaccination with *knowlesi* merozoites with FCA induced some degree of protection (see p. 82) a search for the protective antigens of the merozoite began. Two of the 11 antigens recognized by monkey immune serum were found to be from merozoites.[123] But were these protective and how could sufficient amounts be obtained for vaccination purposes? Sydney Cohen's group at Guy's Hospital, now including Judith Deans and Alan Thomas, elected to apply the recently developed monoclonal antibody techniques to an antigenic analysis of *P. knowlesi* merozoites to identify putative protective antigens and to produce these for vaccination.

In 1982, supported by funds from the MRC and the malaria component of the UNDP/World Bank/ WHO Special Programme for Research and Training in Tropical Diseases, Deans and Thomas prepared two rat monoclonal antibodies that inhibited the *in vitro* multiplication of *P. knowlesi* and both reacted specifically with a single protein of molecular mass (Mr) 66,000.[124] The antigen was processed at the time of red blood cell rupture with merozoite release to give rise to two smaller molecules. Fragments (Fab) of the monoclonal antibody inhibited merozoite invasion and it was postulated that this antigen played a role in merozoite invasion and not in parasite proliferation. Later, it was found using an antiserum prepared against the 66,000 Mr. antigen that it did not prevent merozoites from attaching to erythrocytes, but did inhibit their orientation.[125] Since saponin had been shown to be an effective adjuvant with a vaccine containing whole merozoites Rhesus monkeys were immunized with the purified 66,000 molecular weight antigen with saponin; monkeys produced antibody that inhibited merozoite invasion of red blood cells and four out of six monkeys vaccinated with the purified antigen were protected.[126] It was assumed that where immunization failed to protect it was due to a waning of antibody titer.

The monoclonal antibodies Thomas and Deans generated could have been a tool to isolate the gene encoding the knowlesi antigen (named Pk66), however, before this could be accomplished the group at WEHI (Walter and Eliza Institute) in Melbourne, Australia, published on the molecule from *P. falciparum*.[127]

WEHI was established in 1915 and its principal focus has been immunology, immunopathology, transplantation biology, and virology. In the mid-1970s, Graham Mitchell (b. 1941), an immunologist who had turned his attention to the study of host–parasite interactions, established an Immunoparasitology Unit at WEHI. By 1980, investigations on the molecular biology of malaria under the direction of David Kemp (1945–2013) had begun. Kemp obtained a Ph.D. (1973) from the University of Adelaide in biochemistry. In a time before recombinant DNA techniques had been fully developed he purified feather keratin messenger RNA (mRNA) using nucleic acid hybridization techniques. In 1976 Kemp went to Stanford University to study with David S. Hogness, a leading expert in the study of gene regulation in bacteriophage, and who had recently started using this expertise to study *Drosophila*. Kemp's project was to isolate developmentally regulated genes and this involved construction and analysis of cDNA libraries. In 1978 Kemp returned to Australia and joined WEHI starting as a Research Fellow working on immunoglobulin genes. In 1979 he joined the Parasitology Program at WEHI. Kemp and his colleague Robin Anders (b. 1940) spent the next two years developing a system for cloning malaria antigens. The goal of cloning malaria genes was to try to make a vaccine and the approach used was to identify *P. falciparum* genes critical to immunity. Work on *P. falciparum* was hampered by the small-scale and low yield of parasites from the Trager–Jensen cultures and the inefficiency of enzymes such as reverse transcriptase and terminal transferase, incredibly valuable and difficult to come by reagents that at that time could be obtained from only one laboratory in the world. Malaria parasites had to be cultured continuously for months to harvest enough parasites to allow a single cDNA synthesis to be performed. Although a malaria cDNA library was available by 1982, progress was slow since the vector used, pBR322 expressed antigens in very small amounts. Indeed, the only way to detect expression was to use the incredible sensitivity of the mouse immune system: random lysates of clones from the library were injected and antibody production to malaria antigens assessed. These studies led to the identification of a schizont antigen, however, such methods did not provide a great enough throughput for a meaningful attack on the repertoire of important protective antigens. The turning point was the introduction into the laboratory of the bacteriophage vector λgt11 by Robert Saint, a post-doctoral fellow who joined the WEHI group following a stint at Stanford University, where the vector had been developed in the laboratory of Ronald Davis. With all the steps required for construction and screening of cDNA libraries already in place, the group was quickly able to take advantage of the new vector. Expression levels were at least a 1000-fold higher than pBR322 could provide and direct screening of libraries became possible.

I remember hearing of the success of the WEHI approach toward vaccine development at the April 27–29, 1982 Ciba Foundation meeting *Malaria and the Red Cell*. The Ciba Foundation was distinguished for its promotion of international discussion of biomedicine. Best known were its scientific symposia that were held at the Foundation's headquarters at 41 Portland Place, in central London and close to Oxford Circus, Regents Park, Great Portland Street, and Marylebone. The Foundation provided accommodations as well as dining. Regrettably, Ciba no longer exists (it became Novartis) and although 41 Portland Place is still a venue for meetings/conferences since 2008 it no longer provides overnight accommodations. The attendees at the *Malaria and the Red Cell* meeting were the 'movers and shakers' of malaria. A highlight of the meeting was the announcement by Robin Anders of the WEHI group: "with *P. falciparum* purification of individual proteins is hampered by the small amounts of material available. We have attempted to circumvent these problems by using recombinant DNA techniques to express a wide range of antigens from blood stages of *P. falciparum* in *Escherichia coli*."[128]

The approach used was to construct an expression library of *P. falciparum* cDNA sequences, cloned in *E. coli*.[129] The cDNA sequences were inserted into the β-galactosidase gene of an ampicillin-resistant derivative of the temperature-sensitive lysogenic bacteriophage λgt11. About 5% of the resulting clones expressed *P. falciparum* sequences as polypeptides fused to β-galactosidase. Many clones that expressed falciparum antigens were screened *in situ* with antibodies from immune human sera (from Papua New Guinea) that inhibited *P. falciparum* growth *in vitro*. The WEHI workers claimed: "the cloned *P. falciparum* antigens should facilitate new approaches to the identification of potential vaccine molecules."[128]

At WEHI the recombinant clones were also used to raise monospecific sera either by immunization of laboratory animals or by affinity purification on expressing clones. In turn the monospecific antisera were used to define properties of the corresponding malaria protein. The requirement for affinity-purified serum was circumvented by Anders development of methods for screening using individual sera. This allowed comparisons between exposed individuals who differed in their level of immunity to malaria. Clones expressing many defined malaria proteins were defined by these studies.

In retrospect, it became clear that the screening approach used by the WEHI group, although particularly good at identifying repetitive antigens and proteins containing linear epitopes, was much less efficient at identifying the important subgroup of cysteine-rich proteins. Successful at identifying merozoite antigens such as apical membrane antigen 1 (AMA-1) and MSP, the approach proved incapable of identifying the surface molecule responsible for antigenic variation *P. falciparum* erythrocyte membrane protein 1 (PfEMP1), and the family of merozoite reticulocyte-binding proteins. Working as they were at the beginning of the molecular biology/biotechnology revolution the WEHI group was one of the first to encounter the complexities involved in commercialization of basic research and struggled with the resulting problems of direction and management that come from large scale funding of big science projects, a failure to understand the regulatory requirements, as well as the complexities of bringing a recombinant protein formulation to market. Nonetheless, the technological contribution of the WEHI group was enormous and by building an atmosphere of excitement and optimism about malaria research it attracted a new generation of talented scientists. The work at WEHI ushered in molecular biology studies on malaria — work that continues to this day under the direction of Alan Cowman.

Alan Cowman (b. 1954) began his Ph.D. at WEHI with David Kemp as supervisor in 1980. At the time Kemp was working on immunoglobulin genes and Cowman's project was to analyze the structure of Cμ immunoglobulin transcripts in T cells. This involved making cDNA libraries. Because the Kemp laboratory was very close to those of Robin Anders who had spent more than a decade in Papua New Guinea (and there already was an affiliation of WEHI with the Papua New Guinea Institute of Medical Research for work on malaria), Kemp became interested in blood parasites (malaria and babesiosis) and convinced Cowman to start a Ph.D. on *Babesia bovis*. Together, Kemp and Cowman started working on expression of cDNAs in *E.coli* for ultimately screening sera from humans (in the case of malaria) or *B. bovis* (in the case of cows). During this time they worked out how to express parasite proteins in *E.coli* as β-galactosidase fusion proteins that were screened for antigens using sera. This was the first step into malaria. Cowman wrote his Ph.D. thesis on *B.bovis* (1984) and then started working full time on malaria. As a post-doctoral his first project was to sequence two S-antigen genes from different strains of *P. falciparum*. This resulted in a manuscript published in *Cell*.[130] A second project, finished first, was identification of RESA[131] and this was his first "first author" paper on malaria. Cowman then did a post-doctoral on *Drosophila* with Gerald Rubin at UC Berkeley. In 1987 he returned to WEHI and began working again on malaria and decided to concentrate on drug resistance genes. The main reason he did that was because he was keen to look at transfection of *P. falciparum* and wanted genes that could be used as selectable markers. This led to the identification of the genes for DHFR and DHPS. In subsequent years Cowman and his group have investigated the proteins and protein trafficking routes involved in the remodeling of the falciparum-infected red blood cell, and studied the mechanisms that lead to malaria pathology as well as the identification of merozoite antigens that might serve as the basis for a protective malaria vaccine.

AMA-1 is a micronemal protein that is involved in the reorientation of the merozoite upon contact with the red blood cell and then in the invasion process.[132] Since it has been impossible to delete ("knockout") the gene for AMA-1 it is presumed to be critical for parasite survival. The complete amino acid sequence of AMA-1 from several strains of *P. falciparum* has been determined. Antibody levels to AMA-1 are higher in human populations exposed to natural malaria infections than most other antigens including MSP-1 and the prevalence of such antibodies increases with age of the individual. Therefore, AMA-1 has been considered to have potential as a vaccine candidate. However, with the finding (in 1990) that the AMA-1 gene is polymorphic (i.e. different strains may have up to 100 different amino acid sequences) producing different shaped or sized forms of AMA-1 "has tempered expectations in terms of vaccine-induced broad protective immunity."[133]

There have been several published reports on Phase 1 (safety, immunogenicity and efficacy in a non-endemic setting) vaccine trials with AMA-1 as an *E. coli* produced protein with the adjuvant Montanide ISA720 (containing squalene a metabolizable oil). There were no adverse effects with increasing dosages of 5, 20, 80 μg given intramuscularly at 0, 3, and 6 months, however it showed poor immunogenicity in 6 out of 29 subjects suggesting a loss of potency.[134] In another study with "Combination 1" containing the AMA-1 protein produced in the yeast *Pichia pastoris* and adsorbed to Alhydrogel and with similar dose and schedule it was also well tolerated but again immunogenicity occurred in only 4 out of 22 subjects.[135] In a recent trial the malaria vaccine FMP2.1/ASO2A consisting of a recombinant protein based on AMA-1 with the GSK proprietary adjuvant ASO2 (an oil in water emulsion with deacylated monophosphoryl lipid A and QS21, a saponin agent derived from the soap bark tree *Quillaja saponaria*) was found to be safe and immunogenic when tested in a Phase 1and Phase 2 trial (safety, immunogenicity and efficacy determination of dosage in an endemic setting) in children in Mali, West Africa with doses of 25 μg and 50 μg at 0, 1, and 2 month intervals. The sera inhibited parasite growth *in vitro*.[136] As of this time there is no surrogate measure for protection by a malaria vaccine other than testing in human subjects; this continues to hamper evaluation of vaccine responses. The authors of the Phase 1 and Phase 2 trial sagely concluded: "although these results (with AMA-1) are promising until a blood stage vaccine demonstrates clinical efficacy, immune correlates of vaccine induced protection and the choice of immunogencity endpoints for clinical development decisions will remain a matter of reasoned conjecture."[136]

It is likely that the efficacy of an AMA-1 vaccine will be restricted due to its many forms, however, some malariologists are optimistic that this will not preclude protective effects since "crucial conserved epitopes exist, the function of which can be blocked by antibody."[133] Indeed, it has recently been possible to design three diversity-covering sequences of PfAMA-1 that incorporate 97% of the variability observed in several isolates.[133] When rabbits were immunized with this preparation they produced antibodies that were able to inhibit the *in vitro* growth of three strains of *P. falciparum* (FVO, 3D7 and HB3) from different geographic areas. This suggests that the diversity of AMA-1 was adequately covered, and there is the possibility such a preparation could serve as a protective vaccine. In a more recent study[137] immunization of mice with AMA-1 resulted in sterile immunity in 80% of mice challenged with *P. yoelii* sporozoites. Whether, AMA-1will pass muster in human trials remains undetermined. There are two other caveats in the use of PfAMA-1 as a vaccine: vaccination with AMA-1 might induce the parasite to switch its antigens, and a more effective adjuvant will be required before it can serve as a practical protective vaccine.

v. PfRH5

PfRH5, originally identified by analyzing the *P. falciparum* genome sequence,[138] is located in the rhoptries and is secreted onto the merozoite surface prior to red blood cell invasion. It binds to the Ok blood group antigen, basigin, on the red blood cell surface.[139] The gene for PfRH5, located on chromosome 4, appears to be essential in that it is refractory to genetic deletion i.e. it cannot be 'knocked out.' PfRH5 is a promising vaccine candidate (unlike AMA-1) in that it has limited antigenic diversity.

A full-length recombinant PfRH5 induced antibodies in rabbits and mice that were cross-inhibitory between isolates and inhibited the *in vitro* growth of various *P. falciparum* isolates.[140,141] Humans living in areas where *P. falciparum* is endemic develop anti-PfRH5 antibodies and in Papua New Guinea children with high titer PfRH5 antibodies showed a strong association with protection from symptomatic malaria and high levels of blood parasites were not found; the latter is consistent with the antibodies blocking merozoite invasion. A time to reinfection study in Mali showed that the presence of PfRH5 antibodies was strongly associated with malaria episodes. And, studies in Africa have shown that anti-PfRH5 antibodies and affinity purified human anti-PfRH5 antibodies block merozoite invasion.[142]

A PfRH5 vaccine trial with *Aotus* monkeys infected with *P. falciparum* showed that immunization was protective.[143] All animals immunized with FCA controlled an intravenous challenge with 10^4 parasitized red blood cells, required no antimalarial drug treatment, and 70% of the monkeys immunized were able to resist challenge when PfRH5 was delivered via an adenovirus/pox virus platform previously used in a Phase 1/Ia clinical trial in humans (see Chapter 13). "The optimization of PfRH5 vaccine formulations to achieve and maintain the highest possible levels of antibody will be a major focus of human clinical trials."[143]

It has recently been discovered that PfRH5 has two protein partners involved in merozoite invasion. Monoclonal antibodies against one partner, CyRPA, inhibited *P. falciparum* growth in a passive immunoprotection model.[144] Although CyRPA, and the other protein partner, *P. falciparum* RH5-interacting protein (PfRipr),[145] are essential to invasion neither has a direct role in attachment to the red cell surface rather they serve to secure PfRH5 to the merozoite surface.[141]

Using a single merozoite antigen as a protective vaccine would likely generate an antibody response that would redirect invasion to another pathway and thus evade the immune response. To circumvent this a combination of PfRH and EBA proteins as a multi-component vaccine might induce a broad antibody response sufficient to overcome multiple invasion pathways and thus block merozoite invasion across the *P. falciparum* population.[146] To date no such combination has been tested for efficacy.

vi. A Failed Promise, SPf66

In 1987, with his announcement that he had developed the first synthetic vaccine, the Colombian physician Manuel Elkin Patarroyo stunned the scientific community.[147] He said he had protected monkeys from malaria and now was beginning to test his vaccine on thousands of his countrymen. Patarroyo could have tried several approaches in the development of a protective vaccine i.e. identify the proteins recognized by immune sera, measure the T lymphocyte responses in infected populations to antigens identified by other means (such as antibody), and identify the proteins on the surface of the merozoite or the infected red blood cell. Patarroyo, however, used none of these approaches but directly identified antigens of asexual stage parasites that would protect monkeys against a fatal falciparum infection using a synthesized 45-amino acid peptide as the vaccine.

Working in labs housed in three Victorian-era hospital buildings in Bogota and financed by a series of Colombian presidents the strong-willed and flamboyant Patarroyo seemed to have done what no one else had been able to: make a polymer consisting of three peptides from the merozoite surface, including MSP-1, and then with a deft stroke of legerdemain linked these using a peptide from the sporozoite surface.[148] Patarroyo, after a short period of training at The Rockefeller University with Bruce Merrifield (who in 1984 received the Nobel prize for his "development of methodology for chemical synthesis (of peptides) on a solid matrix") was leading a team 60 scientists, — chemists, molecular biologists, and computer scientists — that had prepared a multi-antigenic, multistage synthetic peptide vaccine, named SPf66. Initially, SPf66 was reported to be able to protect four out of eight *Aotus* monkeys. After repeating the monkey work several times with larger groups of animals he was planning to go forward with humans.[149] This leap forward to human trials was undertaken despite the fact that Socrates Herrera, a former student of Patarroyo, was unable to replicate the work and the Centers for Disease Control (CDC, Atlanta, GA), at the request of WHO, had tested two preparations in *Aotus* monkeys and found an inconsistent immune response and a lack of protection against challenge. Patarroyo in response claimed the CDC had failed to couple the peptides properly!

In 1988, in a preliminary trial with human volunteers, Patarroyo claimed that two out of the five immunized volunteers were protected. In a field trial involving 1,548 human volunteers in Colombia the overall protection rate was reported to be 39%, and in adults was 67% with immunity lasting one to three years.[150,151] Patarroyo was not interested in why the vaccine worked: he simply held news conferences. Like Rumpelstiltskin, the little man in the Grimm brothers fairy tale who could spin straw into gold, Patarroyo with a twinkle in his eye and a smile of satisfaction on his lips showed the assembled reporters a jar of the new vaccine and boasted that the "three series dose costs 30 cents and that's less than the price of Coca-Cola. It's a chemical product, it's completely reproducible, and it's completely pure. There is no possibility of mutation."[148]

Patarroyo was hailed by some as a modern Louis Pasteur and was received as if he were a rock star. By 1993 SPf66 had been tested on 41,000 people in Brazil, Colombia, Ecuador, and Venezuela, where it was claimed the vaccine gave 40–60% efficacy. Critics charged these field trials had been faulty in design.[152] The trials in South America had not included a placebo control, the identities of those immunized with SPf66 were not hidden from the vaccinators, and those who had received the vaccine knew they were not getting a placebo. A further concern was that no one outside of Patarroyo's group had examined the data in his laboratory notebooks.

Trager, on the other hand, defended Patarroyo's work. He wrote to *Science* magazine. "If Manuel Patarroyo's work had been received with less criticism and more cooperation, perhaps we would be five years ahead of where we are now. By the use of the methods of Bruce Merrifield for peptde synthesis — done at the Rockefeller University — a creative young scientist applied these methods to a major medical problem in his country. With support from his government, excellent laboratory facilities and lots of drive and motivation ... He came up wth a combination of three peptides that together gave protection in monkeys. He then did something both clever and original — he took small fragments of these peptides and polymerized them into a synthetic polypeptide. There was accordingly no need for him to use a carrier protein (the method others were using). In his first trials in humans he showed great courage. He chose a cutoff point for treatment that turned out to be safe, yet provided for a significant result."[153]

Buoyed by Trager's endorsement and undeterred by the critics, Patarroyo donated a license for SPf66 to WHO and WHO responded by backing field trials. In a 1994 field trial, backed by the Swiss Tropical Institute, in Tanzania with 586 children vaccinated, the incidence of disease was reduced by 31% — falling far short of earlier claims of much higher efficacy.[154,155] In a 1993–1995 U.S. Army sponsored trial among 1200 children in Thailand, said to be the most expensive ($1.5 million) and the best designed to date there was no efficacy whatsoever. In another trial supported by the MRC and held in The Gambia, 630 infants (6–11 months in age) were immunized with three injections but the vaccine had little effect on protection against first or second attacks of malaria and a delay or prevention of malaria was seen in only 8% of those vaccinated. During a second year follow up there was no significant protection.[156] In 1999 Acosta *et al.* wrote: "given the modest protection previously documented in older age groups and the lack of efficacy in younger infants this vaccine in its current alum-based formulation does not appear to have a role in malaria control in sub-Saharan Africa."[157]

vii. MSP-3

As a graduate student at Northwestern University I came across a publication by the Sergent brothers Etienne and Edmund, who were working at the Pasteur Institute in Algeria carrying out studies to control the transmission of malaria by mosquitoes. But, they did more. They were able to show that chickens were immune to a second attack of the bird malaria *P. gallinaceum* as long the birds had a latent blood infection, whereas upon complete recovery the chickens could become infected. Resistance to reinfection, called premunition, was found to persist for more than two years. Following on their work I tested their findings on premunition with chickens that had recovered from a *P. lophurae* infection, and which were now immune. (I based this on the fact that attempts to induce an infection by intravenous inoculation of large amounts of infected blood produced no apparent infection, and the introduced red blood cells were cleared from the circulation almost immediately). Did the immune birds harbor small numbers of parasites albeit unable to be seen in blood smears? To test for this I injected a large volume of blood from one of these immune birds into very young (and highly susceptible) chicks, and much to my surprise they soon came down with a low-grade blood infection. Evidently the recovered chickens with which I was working showed immunity due to premunition. From my reading of the literature I knew that humans who had recovered from malaria also showed premunition, however this line of research was not pursued by me because not only was the successful *in vitro* culture of *P. falciparum* decades away I was unable to study immunity in human subjects.

In regions where malaria is endemic, humans after surviving many attacks become immune i.e. resist reinfection and show no signs of disease. As demonstrated by McGregor and Cohen (see p. 78) this resistance is due to presence of immunoglobulin. Perhaps, mused Pierre Druilhe, resistance might also be dependent on premunition.

Druilhe (b. 1946), born and educated in Paris, France (MD) and with post-graduate degrees in hematology and medical parasitology (1972), and immunology (1975). In September 2011 Druilhe founded the company Vac-4-All with the aim of capitalizing on 25 years of experience in malaria research, including pre-clinical work and clinical trials. He is a Consultant Tropical Medicine Physician, and works as the Director of the Malaria Vaccine Development Laboratory at the Institut Pasteur, Paris. As an immunologist/parasitologist he revels in the fact that he has marched to the beat of a different drummer. Rather than employing the more traditional methods of moving from bench experiments and then using the mouse immune system to screen for putative protective antigens he began to analyze serum from immune adult Africans (in a state of premunition!) for clinical protection and for identification of potential protective antigens for vaccine development.[158,159]

In the early 1980s Druilhe had obtained sera from immune Africans, however when tested in the laboratory he found the sera did not inhibit the *in vitro* growth of *P. falciparum*. But, laboratory experiments with monocytes from immune Africans were shown to be able to ingest merozoites at a greater rate and this was dependent on the level of specific immunity.[160] Further, passive transfer of antibody from immune adult Africans (in a state of premunition) into infected subjects reduced the severity of their blood infections. Druilhe reasoned: "since immune IgG has proved to be more effective *in vivo* than *in vitro*, its effectiveness may be related to the involvement of other components of the immune system ... Indeed it has been shown ... that ... monocytes are involved in the clearance of ... merozoites after being armed *in vivo* or *in vitro* by IgG from immune individuals."[161] He then did the 'logical' experiment: "a study of the cooperation between normal monocytes and malarial antibodies on *in vitro* proliferation of *P. falciparum* in comparison to the effect of antibodies alone."[162] Laboratory studies showed that immune serum acted indirectly to kill parasites in an antibody-dependent cellular inhibition (ADCI) involving white blood cells, specifically the monocytes. The ADCI mechanism involved two of the seven antibody classes (IgG_1 and IgG_3) as well as secretion of active materials from the monocyte, which at a distance were able to kill parasites within red blood cells. The clinically effective IgGs were purified; using the ADCI mechanism the purified IgG was used to screen a *P. falciparum* expression library. The IgG identified a protein of 48 kDa that localized to the merozoite surface. The protein was named MSP-3[163] and the gene fragment showed no polymorphism. Recombinant proteins and synthetic peptides were then made. Antibodies against the peptides made in mice and human antibodies immunopurified on the peptide were shown to inhibit *P. falciparum* growth in the ADCI assay. The C-terminus domain of MSP-3 was highly conserved among various *P. falciparum* field isolates from Africa and Asia. And, numerous immune-epidemiological studies have consistently shown a strong association between antibodies to MSP-3 of the two classes cooperating in the ADCI mechanism, and with clinical protection. A 96 amino acid region from the C-terminus, a long synthetic peptide (LSP), was used as a subunit vaccine.[164] (It excluded a region having a regulatory role i.e. in that it reduces the immune response). And when individuals were vaccinated there was a consistent association between the antibody responses and a reduced risk of clinical malaria. A phase 1a safety study in healthy Swiss volunteers demonstrated that the MSP-3-LSP vaccine with alum as the adjuvant elicited a strong IgG response and was safe, eliciting antibodies in volunteers that proved able to kill malaria parasites by the ADCI mechanism both *in vitro* and *in vivo*. In 2007, 2 phase 1b clinical trials were conducted in a malaria-endemic area in Tanzania and Burkina Faso in children aged 12–24 months. The trial was not designed to measure vaccine efficacy, however the incidence rates of clinical malaria were found to be substantially lower in the groups that received the MSP-3 vaccine.[165] Parenthetically, it should be noted that evidence in favor of a protective role for MSP-3 in *P. vivax* has been obtained however the relevance of antibodies against the recombinant protein remains untested.[166] Currently, MSP-3 is undergoing a large vaccine efficacy trial in humans.

viii. GMZ2

GMZ2, another malaria vaccine candidate, is a recombinant protein produced in the bacterium *Lactococcus lactis*. It consists of conserved fragments of the merozoite surface protein 3 (MSP-3) and a glutamate-rich protein (GLURP).[167] As noted earlier when *P. falciparum* schizonts rupture the infected red blood cell several antigens are released into the culture supernatants (=exoantigens). Some of these antigens bind to the erythrocyte (red blood cell) surface (e.g. EBA-175), others induce antibody and ADCI immune responses. By screening 100,000 clones from a *P. falciparum* genomic expression library with hyperimmune human sera 19 genomic clones were found to react with the antibodies to the exoantigens. When rescreened with a panel of different sera 4 clones reacted, and these were then used for gene isolation.[163] One of the cloned genes encoded a protein with 1,271 amino acids and had a calculated molecular weight of 145,000. The protein was named GLURP for glutamate rich protein since it contains 22% glutamate residues. GLURP is expressed during the liver (EE) and the asexual red blood cell stages of falciparum malaria. $GLURP_{27-500}$ represents the non-repeat region of the protein. Epidemiological studies have shown that individuals living in malaria endemic regions have high titer antibodies to GLURP and these are associated with protection against disease. The rationale for creating a GLURP-MSP-3 chimera was to obtain an immune response against both domains stronger than that of a single component vaccine. The two components of GMZ2 were tested in Europeans in a clinical phase 1a study using LSPs and both promoted antibodies. Later, a GMZ2 hybrid protein, produced in large quantities, was formulated with alum and given as three injections (10, 30, 100 μg) each one month apart in German malaria-naive adults and showed good safety, tolerability, and modest immunogenicity.[168] Another trial in Gabonese adults compared the higher dose (100 μg) to a control (rabies) vaccine; it too was well tolerated and boosted pre-existing immune responses against the vaccine antigen. A third study in African children 1–5 years of age performed well in doses of either 30 μg or 100 μg. The vaccine induced antibodies for ADCI activity with a capacity to control *in vitro* multiplication of geographically diverse *P. falciparum* strains[168] Whether the GMZ2 vaccine will also inhibit parasite multiplication in infected children from different regions of Africa remains to be investigated.

Chapter 9

PfEMP1, pfalhesin, and DBR

After the publication of the Trager–Jensen method for the continuous cultivation of *Plasmodium falciparum* there was increased funding for malaria research from a variety of sources including the NIH, World Health Organization (WHO), and United States Agency for International Development (USAID) and following the money an ever-increasing number of membrane biochemists were attracted to malaria vaccinology. They knew a lot about membranes and I knew very little so I sought help. I spent a summer (1978) at the Marine Biological Laboratory (MBL) in Woods Hole, MA and shared a laboratory with a friend, Leonard Warren (Wistar Institute), who had an interest in the membranes from cancer cells. Together we began looking at the membranes of red blood cells, however, these could not be those of a duckling (and its resident malaria *P. lophurae*) since the MBL devoted to research on marine organisms frowned on the use of terrestrial animals. So we began our work on a marine vertebrate — the dogfish. When the collecting boat came in Len and I gathered up syringes, needles, and flasks, and went down to the dock where we laid out a live dogfish and bled it. This was the source of red blood cell membranes and during that summer I learned a great deal about membrane isolation and characterization. After a stint in University Administration I was back at the laboratory bench and it was fun. After the summer ended, I brought the techniques I learned at the MBL to UCR and my technician successfully applied it to *P. lophurae* and the duckling red blood cell. I also recruited an MD electron microscopist from Japan,

Yuzo Takahashi, and he used cytochemical and immunochemical methods to distinguish the membranes of the parasite and the duckling red blood cell; they were found to be different biochemically and immunologically.[169] The question now became: what was the basis for these changes? Parasite proteins or modified red blood cell membrane proteins? And, more importantly would similar changes be found in the falciparum-infected red blood cell?

After 1976 (and the taming of *P. falciparum*) it became more and more difficult for my laboratory to obtain NIH funding for a model system such as *P. lophurae* and the duckling red cell. Indeed, the NIH (and several other funding agencies) could no longer see any advantage in using bird malaria when there was the real thing — a human *Plasmodium*. It became quite clear my laboratory would have to redirect the research to *P. falciparum* were we to obtain continued extramural funding.

i Knobs and Adhesion

A century ago Amico Bignami (1862–1929) and Giuseppe Bastianelli (1862–1959), working in the Rome laboratory of Batistta Grassi, examined the blood of a farmer working in the malarious area of the Campagna and found the patient's peripheral blood had only ring stage parasites and red blood cells containing gametocytes.[170] Further work showed that the more mature parasite stages, absent from the peripheral blood, were localized in the deep tissues. By this they discovered sequestration in *P. falciparum* i.e. the adhesion of red cells bearing the mature pigment-containing parasites (trophozoites and schizonts) to the endothelial cells that line post-capillary venules of the deep tissues. Although their observations explained why the mature stage malaria parasites were absent from the peripheral blood, whereas the young, unpigmented ring-stage parasites circulated freely in the peripheral blood, it did not reveal the mechanisms for such preferential binding. Much later, the development of transmission and scanning electron microscopes made it possible to describe differences in the red blood cell surface when such cells harbored different developmental stages of *P. falciparum*, and these would provide clues to an understanding of the mechanisms for the differing adhesive properties of the falciparum-infected red blood cell.

Red blood cells bearing the mature stages of *P. falciparum* lose their biconcave disc shape, are distorted, and covered with submicroscopic elevations of the plasma membrane (~100 nm in diameter and ~20 nm in height) underlain by an electron dense plaque, called "knobs."[171] The numbers of knobs per infected red blood cell has been estimated to be as low as 500 or as high as 6,000. By contrast, red blood cells infected with ring-stage parasites have a smooth surface and are knobless. These observations were first made by Trager, Rudzinska, and Bradbury[172] using transmission electron microscopy of blood samples from patients living in Africa and later Luse and Miller found the same knobby structures on red cells from falciparum-infected *Aotus* monkeys.[173] By transmission electron microscopy attachment to blood vessel endothelial cells was seen to be via the knobs.[174] Soon after the successful *in vitro* cultivation of *P. falciparum* Susan Langreth (working in Trager's Rockefeller University laboratory) was able to show that knobs were present in the cultures of red blood cells infected with *P. falciparum*.[175] And in 1981, when Udeinya *et al.*[176] were able to mimic sequestration *in vitro* (called cytoadherence) by binding falciparum-infected red blood cells to endothelial cells (and later C32 amelanotic melanoma cells) and to show that adhesion was at knobs the conclusion was inescapable: knobs mediate adhesion. Additionally, immunocytochemical staining of falciparum-infected with hyperimmune human serum showed that only the knobs were labeled.[177] Thus, it became clear that the changes in the knob were sufficient to be recognized as "non-self" i.e. they were antigenically distinct. These studies (as well as those concerned with schizont-infected cell agglutination (SICA), see below) led to a search by several laboratories for the "non-self" molecules that were the "glue" of the knob. In addition, there was a stated practical goal: identification of the "glue" might be the basis for a protective malaria vaccine.

ii SICA and Antigenic Variation

Neil Brown (1929–2012) was brought up in North London, educated at the Southgate Grammar School and graduated from Imperial College London in 1953. After two years at the London School of Hygiene and Tropical Medicine, he joined May & Baker Ltd., becoming one of the team that subsequently discovered and developed Isomethamedium, used for over 40 years for the treatment of cattle trypanosomiasis in Africa. Resigning from May & Baker, he was recruited by Frank Hawking, Head of Parasitology at the NIMR, to screen for compounds active against trypanosomes and malaria parasites. Finding drug screening extremely tedious, he sought the support of Sir Charles Harrington, Director of the NIMR, for permission to investigate variable antigens of trypanosomes. This was granted for three years. Initially, Neil Brown studied the variable trypanosome antigens, however, when Neil completed his Ph.D. (University of London 1963), and a post became available at the NIMR for screening for a malaria vaccine Neil switched his interests from trypanosomes to malaria. Neil was convinced that the only way to tackle the malaria vaccine problem was to pursue basic research, which he immediately set about doing.

Following the observations of Monroe Eaton,[178] who had shown that serum from monkeys infected with *P. knowlesi* could agglutinate (clump) schizont-infected red blood cells, Neil and his colleague Ivor Brown used the SICA reaction to show that SICA was both species- and stage-specific i.e. it was an antigen on the surface of the infected red blood cell, and relapse parasites from a single isolate differed in their SICA antigens.[179] In a series of seminal papers over the following years, Brown and Brown demonstrated that a chronic *P. knowlesi* malaria infection was maintained by the serial expression of different antigenic types and that immunity to infection was associated with the development of variant-specific antibodies. Brown hypothesized that antigenic variation in malaria resulted from the selection of a minor parasite population, and that the host-produced antibody acted as a signal for the induction of antigenic switching.[180,181] Neil Brown's hypothesis was based on the following experiment: in rhesus monkeys, immunization in Freund's incomplete adjuvant (FIA) with *P. knowlesi* bearing a particular SICA induced high titer antibodies. When immunized or naive monkeys were challenged with 10, 100, or 1,000 *P. knowlesi* expressing the same SICA antigen to which the immunized monkeys had been sensitized, the infections in sensitized or control monkeys were nearly identical in terms of the time at which parasites appeared in the blood, yet the sensitized monkeys contained parasites that were of a different SICA.[182]

When the group at the NIMR discovered that spontaneous relapses were usually well-controlled in the immune host but that the relapse variant was fully virulent on inoculation into non-immune monkeys they suggested there was an additional immunity that was not variant specific.[181] Not only were they able to confirm the observations of Freund, in which monkeys immunized with Freund's complete antigen (FCA) developed an immunity that transcended the parasite's capacity for antigenic variation,[45,179] they also discovered that after vaccination by infection and cure, or by dead parasitized cells in FIA, and then challenged with the same variant, there was an intense but short-lived infection that was eliminated in a few weeks.[182] This immunity did not depend on the presence of a chronic infection and unlike the immunity usually occurring in chronic infections it was effective against other strains of *P. knowlesi*, though not against other monkey malarias (*P. inui* and *P. cynomolgi*).

In addition to the malaria vaccine work at the NIMR, there was another team headed by Sydney Cohen at Guy's Hospital Medical School in London. When Cohen learned of the experiments at the NIMR and read the conclusion to the Brown and Brown report: "this variation can explain the chronicity of the disease and the inconsistent results with artificial vaccines ... Some degree of immunity transcending antigenic variation also occurs, but its potential value as a possible basis for the development of a vaccine is uncertain."[179] Cohen was more than irritated. Indeed, the passive transfer experiments with immune IgG he had carried out with Ian McGregor in The Gambia had raised the hope that a malaria vaccine was possible. To counter the NIMR conclusion Cohen wrote: "despite the wide antigenic variability ... within individual strains of *P. knowlesi* ... the occurrence of cross-immunization between variants is encouraging from the point of view of vaccine production."[183] The challenge ahead was to identify that strain-transcending protective antigen.

Cohen could not accept that parasites could change their antigens, and he went on the offensive, countering Brown's contentions and arguing that even if antigenic variation did occur in *P. knowlesi* it could be downplayed as a special case and was not relevant to the development of a protective vaccine for humans. Neil Brown, however, was the kind of person who would not "bend the knee" to a dismissive peer such as Cohen, despite the latter's eminence as Professor of Chemical Pathology, and Chairman of the Medical Research Council (MRC) Tropical Medicine Research Board, and this led to a serious falling out, and bitter arguments between them persisted for years. But, by the time Neil Brown retired from the NIMR (1994) there was a general recognition of his insight and acknowledgment by his peers. And, Neil Brown's final triumph would come with the genomic era when John Barnwell and coworkers convincingly proved that *P. knowlesi* had the genetic capacity to express successive SICA variants, that the SICA antigens were high molecular weight, polymorphic, parasite-encoded proteins uniformly distributed on the surface of the red blood cell, and that the Rhesus monkey spleen plays a critical role in expression of SICA.[184]

iii. Antigenic Variation and *P. falciparum* Erythrocyte Membrane Protein 1 (PfEMP1)

Antigenic variation (first described for *P. knowlesi*) is now accepted as an important immunologic phenomenon especially as it occurs in falciparum malaria. Further, antigenic switching *in vivo* is an attractive parasite evasion strategy since it does not occur until after the appearance of a specific anti-variant antibody and consequently the malaria parasite makes more efficient use of its variant repertoire. Even more striking, antigenic variation suggests an active signaling process between host and parasite. Antigenic variation is important for an understanding of the nature of *P. falciparum* infections that are chronic, with immunity to infection acquired slowly and rarely, if ever, complete and where severe disease on a per infection basis is rare.

Chris Newbold (b.1952) trained as a biochemist (MA, Ph.D. Cambridge University 1978) joined Neil Brown at the NIMR in 1979 to begin to study the synthesis of the SICA antigens of *P. knowlesi*. Using radioactive amino acids Newbold showed that the parasite synthesized novel antigens some of which appeared to be related to SICA.[185] (SICA had to be of parasite origin because the mature red blood cell is incapable of protein synthesis). After Newbold moved to Oxford University (1984) he continued to work on antigenic variation and when laboratory grown *P. falciparum* became available it was only natural that after identification of the parasite-encoded SICA antigens he would want to see whether similar antigens were present on the surface of *P. falciparum* infected red blood cells, and whether these played a role in sequestration and immune evasion. Newbold now leads the Molecular Parasitology Group at The Weatherall Institute of Molecular Medicine where he continues to work on mechanisms of disease and immune evasion in malaria.

The Australian born Russell J. Howard (b.1950) was also on the hunt for the new antigens on the surface of the malaria-infected red cells. In 1972, Howard received his bachelors' degree in Biochemistry with honors from Melbourne University, Victoria, Australia and the Ph.D. (1975) on the biochemistry of the marine alga *Caulerpa simpliciuscula*. In 1976 Howard began his career in the field of molecular pathogenesis of malaria with post-doctoral studies in the Immunoparasitology Laboratory of Graham F. Mitchell at Walter and Eliza Hall Institute (WEHI). Beginning in 1979 Howard sought to find evidence for the variant surface antigen of *P. falciparum* as a Visiting Associate in the NIH laboratory of Louis Miller in Bethesda, Maryland.

Using radioactive iodine Howard and his NIH colleagues were able to identify a variant protein on the surface of rhesus red blood cells infected with *P. knowlesi*.[186] Later, using similar techniques, and with the collaboration of James H. Leech (1948–1994), and John W. Barnwell, the work was extended to *Aotus* red blood cells infected with *P. falciparum*.[187] Strain-specific antigens could also be labeled with radioactive amino acids indicating they were of parasite origin rather than altered host components. The members of the protein family were variable in molecular size, but had in common several biochemical properties including accessibility to surface radioiodination, detergent solubility, and removal by low concentrations of trypsin. Immunoprecipitation of these proteins with antibody correlated with the capacity of the immune sera to block the adherence of infected red blood cells in a strain-specific fashion.

By 1984 there was evidence that the surface variant protein of *P. falciparum*, now named PfEMP1, was similar to SICA. It could be removed from the surface of falciparum-infected red cells by exposure to low concentrations of the protein-digesting enzyme trypsin and after protein "stripping" the infected red blood cells lost their stickiness. That is, trypsin removed the surface "glue." Sera taken from people immune to one falciparum strain precipitated PfEMP1 from the same strain but not from others. These sera also blocked *P. falciparum*-infected red cell binding to endothelial cells from blood vessels in a strain-specific way. The conclusion was inescapable: the parasite made a protein, PfEMP1, responsible for both blood vessel attachment (sequestration) and antigenic variation i.e. it was the strain-specific "glue." Through switching to different forms of PfEMP1 i.e. "changing its spots" *P. falciparum* is able to evade the host immune system, and by PfEMP1 acting as the "glue" of sequestration passage through the spleen — the graveyard of the red blood cell — is avoided. It has been claimed that antibodies to PfEMP1 are responsible for regulating the parasite density in the blood such that there is a concomitant decrease in the severity of disease, leading to a chronic infection and non-sterilizing immunity. Immunity to PfEMP1 may have other effects: it can influence mosquito transmission by regulating the numbers of asexual blood stages with the potential to become transmission stages (gametocytes) and by directly targeting early gametocytes could prevent their maturation. Since its discovery, PfEMP1 has been considered an attractive vaccine candidate. Indeed, PfEMP1 has been an especially tantalizing target because it is exposed on the surface of the infected red blood cell for ~20 hour and correlations have been found between antibody recognition of it and clinical protection against severe malaria. Based on this it has been hypothesized that vaccination with PfEMP1 might promote an early buildup of immunity in children to the most virulent parasites and significantly reduce malaria-related deaths.

In 1988 Howard left the NIH and created the Laboratory of Infectious Diseases at the DNAX Research Institute of Molecular and Cellular Biology (Palo Alto, CA) where he continued work on antigenic variation in malaria; in 1992 he joined the Affymax Research Institute as Vice President and Director of Cell Biology, and in 1994 became its President and Scientific Director. At Affymax, Howard and colleagues were able to clone and sequence the gene for PfEMP1.[188] The gene for PfEMP1, named var (for variant), was also cloned and sequenced independently by two other laboratories — at Oxford University under the leadership of Chris Newbold[189] and at the NIH[190] under the leadership of Louis Miller. Today, thanks to genome sequence analysis we know the PfEMP1 proteins are coded for by ~60 var (variant) genes.[191,192] The var genes localized primarily to the ends (telomeres) of all 14 chromosomes of *P. falciparum*, are extremely divergent in their DNA sequence, and theoretically could code for very large size proteins (~200,000–500,000 molecular mass).[191,193]

Having succeeded in his personal quest of identifying the var gene, Russell Howard abandoned further research on malaria. In 1996 he became President and Chief Operating Officer of Maxygen during its incubator phase and in 1998 he became its President and Chief Executive Officer. In 2008 he left Maxygen to found Oakbio, a company that designs microbes for production of cost-competitive chemicals using carbon dioxide emissions as a carbon source.

Sequestration and immune evasion are linked to two different adhesive domains of PfEMP1: Duffy binding-like (DBL), and cysteine-rich interdomain region (CIDR); and the molecule contains an acidic region called the acidic terminal sequence (ATS) presumed to anchor the molecule to the red cell surface. The DBLs are grouped into five different varieties: α, β, γ, δ, ε, and the CIDR region can be divided into three different types: α, β, and γ.

Since PfEMP1 is involved in the change from one variant to another (and only one variant is expressed at a time) this challenges the developer of a PfEMP1-based vaccine to make the appropriate choice of a conserved antigen. Several proof-of-principle studies using animal models have provided a modicum of encouragement that such an approach may be feasible. The first immunization study utilized the conserved CIDRα domain responsible for binding to the molecule CD36, present on the surface of cells that line the small blood vessels.[194] A recombinant protein, recombinant cysteine-rich interdomain region1 (rCIDR1) was prepared. The 179 amino acids containing seven cysteine residues of this rCIDR protein were found to constitute the minimal adhesion motif. The recombinant protein blocked adhesion of all the CD36-binding strains that were tested and it was claimed that no matter the CIDR sequence from various isolates the protein could fold into a conserved structure to mediate binding to CD36. Immunization of *Aotus* monkeys with the rCIDR delayed the appearance of blood parasites (FVO strain) and were of the same strain of PfEMP1 used for the preparation of the vaccine, however, the monkeys were not protected against severe infections and to prevent death all animals required treatment with antimalarials. This result differed from a previous study using a less virulent strain (MC) in which monkeys had been protected. The question remains whether immunization with rCIDR will protect against disease.

In follow-up studies, when plasmid DNAs encoding several CIDRα variants[195] or DNA vaccination followed by a boost with three CIDRα recombinant proteins[196] or chimeric proteins produced by shuffling of PfEMP1 genes[197] were used to vaccinate mice cross-reactive antibodies developed. This again suggested the possibility for developing a vaccine able to induce variant transcending immunity, however, whether this regimen would protect *Aotus* (or humans) against challenge remains unknown. Further, it must be borne in mind that because the human responses to DNA vaccines are so different from those of mice the findings may have little practical relevance for developing a PfEMP 1-based vaccine.

Approximately 1% of *P. falciparum* infections result in cerebral malaria (CM), a clinical condition defined as unarousable coma associated with falciparum parasites. Around 90% of CM cases occur in children in sub-Saharan Africa and in adults in South East Asia CM accounts for 50% of deaths. Despite the precise cause of CM being controversial what is indisputable is the presence of sequestered infected red blood cells in the brains of people dying from the disease. The pathogenesis of CM is a multifactorial process, with sequestration, inflammation, and endothelial dysfunction in the microvessels of the brain leading to coma. With regard to sequestration, PfEMP1 binding to the endothelial cells has received the most attention. PfEMP1 binds to more than a dozen molecules including ICAM-1, CD36, and endothelial protein C receptor (EPCR), thrombospondin (TSP) and chondroitin sulfate. Isolates from severe malaria patients and particularly those with CM have a higher binding to ICAM-1 although this is not seen in all studies.[198] However, ICAM-1 is not the only receptor involved in CM pathogenesis.

A recent study[199] found that in severe childhood malaria including CM binding of PfEMP1 was to EPCR via CIDRα1. Indeed, an analysis of 885 CIDRα1 sequences showed that all had a conserved domain of 14 amino acids responsible for binding to EPCR with nanomolar affinities, and using peptides from the EPCR binding region of two different CIDRα1 domains it was possible to purify antibodies from Tanzanian children; these antibodies partially blocked the binding of heterologous CIDRα1 domains and CIDRα1-expressing falciparum infected red cells to EPCR. This study suggests that *P. falciparum* populations have evolved high affinity CIDRα1–EPCR interactions that are not easily broken by human antibody responses specific for genetic polymorphisms. It has been suggested that "while a cocktail vaccine of several CIDRα1 peptides might induce a similar strain transcending immunity another approach to achieve this might be to synthesize a novel peptide that mimics the conserved shape and binding potential of diverse CIDRα1 domains."[200]

Another receptor on microvascular endothelial cells in a variety of tissues but not the brain is CD36 (cluster of differentiation 36). Sequestration in these tissues could promote parasite survival and transmission while minimizing injury and death.[201] Almost all *P. falciparum* lines bind to CD36 found on the surface of platelets, monocytes, dendritic cells as well as endothelial cells. It is generally believed that CD36 provides a stable and long-lasting anchor for the binding of falciparum-infected cells. The CD36 domain responsible for binding the infected red cells has been reported to reside in amino acids 139–184. The CIDR domain involved in binding of falciparum-infected red cells is under strong selection pressure for adhesion to CD36 and it has been suggested that this leads to severe malaria. However, a recent well-designed study did not show a significant association of CD36 variants with malaria severity.[202]

iv. PfEMP1 and Placental Adhesion

Each year over 50 million women are exposed to the risk of malaria during pregnancy. Pregnancy malaria (PM) results in substantial maternal and especially fetal and infant morbidity, causing as many as 200,000 infant deaths annually. Pregnant women are more susceptible to malaria than are non-pregnant women and this susceptibility is greatest during the first and second pregnancies. The only malaria drug currently recommended by the WHO for use during pregnancy is sulfadoxine–pyrimethamine and as with most antimalarials there is the problem of parasite resistance. A vaccine against PM may be an option to prevent illness and death in pregnant women and children. Indeed, because there is reduced susceptibility to PM in women over several pregnancies, it suggests that women are able to develop immunity to PM after infection. Further, women develop broadly reactive antibodies to infected red blood cells isolated from the placenta.

Michal Fried (b.1960) grew up in Israel, received her B.Sc. and M.Sc. from Ben Gurion University of the Negev (1984, 1987 respectively), and then studied the sexual stage antigens of the coccidian parasite *Eimeria maxima* for her Ph.D. at the Hebrew University in Jerusalem (1991). Upon completion of the doctorate, she wanted to continue studying parasitic diseases that impact human health, particularly malaria. After spending three year at NIH studying malaria (with David Kaslow and where she met Patrick Duffy) she had the opportunity to visit and carry out research in Kenya (dreams do come true!). In the process of designing a study on malaria pathogenesis she read articles on the impact of PM on both the mother and her baby, and around that time heard a lecture from Robert Desowitz describing the complications associated with PM. Despite the large number of publications describing the outcomes associated with this syndrome, it remained unclear why pregnant women were more susceptible to malaria. In the belief that a better understanding of the disease might help in the development of interventions Michal set her sights on uncovering the molecular basis responsible for the syndrome.

Parasite sequestration in the placenta was described by a number of studies more than a century ago, however, only in 1958 did Cannon note the association between parity and the frequency of malaria infection during pregnancy. In succeeding years, other studies confirmed these observations. It was assumed that the increased susceptibility to PM was due to pregnancy-related immunosuppression, however this did not explain the differences seen between first and later pregnancies. An alternative hypothesis to this model was developed as a result of a study begun in 1995 by Fried and her colleague Patrick Duffy i.e. the placenta presents new receptors for parasite adhesion. This landmark study described the unique binding of placental parasites to chondroitin sulfate A (CSA), a molecule expressed on the surface of placental cells. Because CSA is not readily accessible for parasite adhesion in the non-pregnant female, primigravid women are naive to this parasite subpopulation. In subsequent years, this work was extended to show that with successive pregnancies, women develop immunity to placental parasites.

The possibility for a specific vaccine for pregnant women was unthinkable prior to the discovery of antibodies to placental parasites able to block parasite adhesion to CSA and leading to reduced infection rates and lower parasite densities, however, over the past decade all that has changed. There is now not only increased funding (especially by the Bill & Melinda Gates Foundation) there is also an increased awareness of the problem by governmental organizations.

Michal believes the key ingredients to developing a PM vaccine are a better understanding of disease pathogenesis and identification of the protective immune responses rather than a simple association between antibody levels to specific antigens and a reduction in disease severity. The latter may only indicate exposure/experience, not necessarily protective immune responses. Guided by these factors, together with the availability of advanced technologies as well as generous funding she is optimistic a pregnancy vaccine will be developed. Currently, Fried and Duffy, as well as several other groups are working on developing a PM vaccine.

Adhesion studies have shown that the parasitized erythrocytes from the placenta predominantly bind to the glycosaminoglycan (GAG) CSA, whereas infected red blood cells from the peripheral blood of pregnant women bind to other receptors, primarily CD36. Such findings suggest either that the placenta secretes a factor or there are serum-specific factors present only during pregnancy and these "turn on" parasite genes that allow binding to the placenta. The placenta, in turn, has a unique set of high affinity adhesion receptors for binding the rare CSA-binding malaria-infected red blood cells and these preferentially transcribe the var2csa gene, a member of the PfEMP1 family (see above). Transcription of var2csa is upregulated in parasites selected to bind to CSA and this gene is semi-conserved between geographically diverse isolates. The var2csa gene encodes DBL domains that bind CSA *in vitro* and in Malawian women var2csa predominates. An interesting observation is that CSA binding lines are phagocytized at significantly lower levels than CD36 binding lines and when the parasites are engineered to lose the var2csa gene (i.e. "knocked out") the red blood cells have impaired placental adhesion and lose the ability to adhere to CSA.

Currently, var2csa is a leading vaccine candidate for PM. Var2csa has a high molecular mass and contains six DBL domains. This has complicated manufacture of the full-length protein for vaccine development. Therefore, the goal of a PM vaccine has been to identify the best domain combination as an alternative to the full-length protein.[203] It has been shown that most single domain antigens, save for DBL4 and DBL5 have limited adhesion blocking activity. When antibodies were generated to these domains (expressed in *E.coli*) it was possible to inhibit the binding of maternal infected red cells to the placental tissue in a manner comparable to plasma collected from multigravid women.[204] More recent studies suggested that CSA-binding epitopes are located in the N-terminal region of var2csa, and antibodies raised against recombinant proteins derived from that region (NTS-DBL2) elicited functional anti-adhesion antibodies.[205] As the authors of this report state: "these results are a promising step forward for vaccine development." Currently there are two products that will go into a Phase 1 study, one in Copenhagen and the other from INSERM (France) which will be tested in Burkina Faso. The vaccine products are designed based on the earlier work that showed the association between naturally acquired anti-adhesion antibodies and improved pregnancy outcome.

A PM vaccine would specifically target the parasitized red cells sequestering in the placenta. Such a vaccine could be given to young women before their first pregnancy and would be aimed at inducing high levels of the PM-specific antigens generally seen in the women after successive pregnancies and who become resistant to PM. Ideally, such a vaccine would result in protection against maternal anemia, pre-term delivery and fetal growth restriction, but would leave unaffected those parasites that do not express the non-pregnancy associated malaria PfEMP1 and thus would be of little benefit to the child.

v. Pfalhesin and DBR

In 1976, the WHO established The Special Programme for Research and Training in Tropical Diseases (TDR) with a mission to promote scientific collaboration and to help coordinate, support, and influence global efforts to combat a portfolio of major diseases of the poor and disadvantaged, including malaria. Scientists and public health experts were brought together to help set the Programme's overall research priorities and goals. The operations of TDR would be (and were) overseen by specialized Scientific Working Groups (SWGs), each led by a Steering Committee, one of which was the Chemotherapy of Malaria (CHEMAL). In 1976 I became a member of CHEMAL. CHEMAL met twice a year. Most of the meetings were in Geneva, Switzerland at WHO headquarter but we also met in Belem, Brazil, Lucknow, India, Panama, Bangkok, Thailand, Basle, Switzerland, New York City, and Washington, DC. At these meetings grant proposals were critically reviewed and funding awards made.

During one of my trips to Geneva for CHEMAL I met a young biochemist, Jean Gruenberg, and I invited him to join my laboratory and extend his studies on transport in trypanosomes to malaria. When he arrived he decided not to work on membrane transport. Rather, in collaboration with a graduate student, David Allred, they studied the dynamics of knob formation by scanning and transmission electron microscopy as well as biochemistry.[171,206] Using a clever membrane stripping technique and radioactive labeling no evidence was found for the insertion of parasite proteins into the red blood cell membrane. This put us at odds with those laboratories studying antigenic variation (especially those of Newbold and Howard) since at the time the prevailing notion was that parasite-encoded proteins of the knob, particularly PfEMP1, was exclusively responsible for both antigenic variation and sequestration. Indeed, the rivalry between these groups and our own led to their disregard of our published work on cytoadherence.

Prior to 1995 our laboratory (as well as others) attempted, using conventional biochemical techniques, to isolate the parasite-encoded proteins inserted into the red cell membrane of cells infected with *P. falciparum*. Indeed, in 1986 during a sabbatical at the WEHI in Melbourne, Australia I decided to try isolating this protein by using radioactive iodine to label the surface of infected red blood cells, allowing these to bind to endothelial cells, and then by collecting the high binders expected to have enriched PfEMP1 sufficiently so it could be isolated by conventional biochemistry. It was quickly found (by my technician who carried out the binding studies) that the iodinated cells did not bind. This suggested the possibility that the surface iodinated proteins did not play a role in adhesion. This fruitless sabbatical leave convinced me that PfEMP1 was not on the surface or even if it were there it was not the only molecule responsible for adhesion. Indeed, these results and our inability to find evidence for the insertion of parasite-encoded proteins in *P. falciparum* infected red cells (based on the work of David Allred and Jean Gruenberg) led us to suggest that in addition to plasmodial proteins the malaria parasite might alter the red blood cell surface by a modification of intrinsic red blood cell membrane proteins. In this notion we were not alone.

At the 1982 Ciba Symposium *Malaria and the Red Cell* (a Symposium suggested by Neil Brown!) Russell Howard had formulated a similar hypothesis stating: "some component of the knob mediates binding to endothelial cells. Support comes from IgG in homologous immune serum that inhibits or reverses binding of *P. falciparum* infected cells to cultured endothelial cells *in vitro*. Knobs must contain other components, however, besides those required for endothelial attachment and these should be elucidated as monoclonal antibodies become available." He went on: "new antigens in the surface membrane of infected erythrocytes could arise by insertion of parasite-derived proteins, glycoproteins or glycolipids. Alternatively, host membrane components could be altered in structure or arrangement, for example, by limited proteolysis or by forming new protein–protein complexes to create new antigenic determinants for the surface of the infected red cell. Again we can predict that our understanding of the role of these altered host antigens in antimalaria immunity will become clearer when monoclonal antibodies are available."[207]

In 1985, a graduate student in my laboratory, Enrique Winograd, whom I had met during my attendance at a 1984 scientific meeting in Bogota, Colombia was able to produce a monoclonal antibody to the surface of live *P. falciparum* infected red blood cells, thanks to the collaboration of a UCR colleague in the Plant Pathology Department, David Gumpf, with expertise in producing monoclonal antibodies against citrus viruses. By immunoelectron and immunofluorescence microscopy this monoclonal antibody localized to the knobby surface of the falciparum-infected red cells and was able to prevent adhesion to target cells i.e. they were cytoadherence-blockers. Using Western blotting, immunoprecipitation and peptide mapping of the surface of iodinated red cells it was determined that the antibody did not recognize a parasite encoded protein, but instead an intrinsic membrane protein, the anion transporter, named band 3, albeit in an altered form.[208]

Band 3 is ~95 kDa membrane spanning protein tetramer and is the most abundant red blood cell membrane protein with a million copies per red blood cell. In collaboration with a post-doctoral fellow in my laboratory, Ian Crandall, the amino acid sequence of band 3 that contributed to the antigenic change was identified using peptide scanning against a battery of monoclonal antibodies he had produced. Once we had the amino acid sequence in hand we decided to have various peptide sequences synthesized. When I suggested to Crandall that he test the peptides for anti-adhesive activity I was not optimistic. Surprisingly, peptides with the amino acid sequence HPLQKTY (= histidine–proline–leucine–glutamine–lysine–threonine–tyrosine and corresponding to residues 546–553 of the band 3 protein) blocked adhesion of infected red cells *in vitro*, as did antibodies to the synthetic peptides and if the sequences of amino acids in the peptide were scrambled there was no anti-adhesive effect.[209] We named the HPLQKTY peptide, pfalhesin. In collaboration with Jurg Gysin (in France) and Bill Collins (at the CDC) these synthetic peptides were infused into *Saimiri* and *Aotus* monkeys infected with *P. falciparum* and there was a flood of mature parasites into the circulation because (we theorized) the peptide blocked the sites for infected red cell adherence.[210] In collaboration with other investigators serum from those living in an endemic area (and who were immune to malaria and were not anemic) specifically reacted with the synthetic peptides.[211] Neil Guthrie another post-doctoral in my lab was able to coat polystyrene beads with the peptides and these pfalhesin-coated beads behaved as if they were knobby infected red cells.[212] Clearly, pfalhesin was a contributing factor for the adhesion of the falciparum-infected red blood cell.

Subsequent to the work on pfalhesin we used the anion transport inhibitor DIDS (4, 4′ diisothiocyano-2, 2′-stilbenesulfonic acid) to block the adhesion of falciparum-infected blood cells to amelanotic melanoma cells. In human red cells DIDS binding occurs in a region close to the HPLQKTY sequence, namely YETFSKLIKIFQDH (= tyrosine–glutamic acid–threonine–phenylalanine–serine–lysine–leucine–isoleucine–lysine–isoleucine–phenylalanine–glutamine–aspartic acid–histidine corresponding to residues 537–547 of the band 3 protein). Synthetic peptides with this sequence (called the DIDS binding region, DBR) and antibodies prepared in chickens and rabbits against this sequence were found to block adhesion.[213] Sera obtained from individuals living in an endemic region for malaria — so-called "immune sera" — were shown to contain antibodies to the DIDS-binding region peptide. We hypothesized that both the DIDS-binding region and pfalhesin were cryptic in the uninfected red blood cell but upon infection with *P. falciparum* these amino acid sequences became exposed due to a clustering of band 3. Further, we were able to demonstrate band 3 clustering and binding of autologous IgG by treatment of uninfected human red blood cells with agents known to cluster the band 3 protein e.g. acridine orange, BS^3, $ZnCl_2$.[213] In another study we were able to show that oxidative stress (by exposure to t-butylhydroperoxide) results in band 3 clustering and exposure of the DBR. And, when band 3 clustering was induced in uninfected red cells by treatment with acridine orange it exposed a cryptic tryptic cleavage site (presumably close to residues 551 and/or 562 of band 3 protein); when such cells were treated with trypsin there was cleavage of band 3 (reminiscent of the removal of PfEMP1 by trypsin).[214]

Our findings were considered by some investigators of sequestration and PfEMP1 to be in opposition to their work and to minimize the possibility of PfEMP1 serving as a vaccine candidate. Occasionally this led to face-to-face confrontations at scientific meetings and possibly it affected peer review as well as jeopardizing research funding. It should be categorically stated that PfEMP1 and pfalhesin/DBR are not identical. The exposed band 3 peptide sequences are neither isolate specific nor are they parasite-encoded, but the DBR sequence and PfEMP1 do have a common receptor, CD36. And, pfalhesin also binds to TSP, which is not a receptor for PfEMP1. Based on the available evidence I hypothesized that at a minimum the adhesion of *P. falciparum*-infected red blood cells is mediated by a combination of parasite-encoded proteins such as PfEMP1, and exposed amino acid sequences in band 3 protein. These studies have clearly shown that surface membrane modifications of falciparum-infected red blood cells involved in adhesion need not involve solely parasite-encoded proteins. However, a metabolically active parasite is essential to promote the observed membrane alterations i.e. conformational change and exposure of a cryptic amino acid sequence of band 3 protein.

With regard to the relevance of pfalhesin/DBR to a possible malaria vaccine we have shown:

(1) The microvascular endothelial receptors for the peptides HPLQKTY and YETFSKLIKIFQDH are the type 3 repeat of TSP and CD36, respectively.

(2) (a) Infusion of HPLQKTY into falciparum infected *Aotus* and *Saimiri* monkeys leads to a block in sequestration and accumulation in the peripheral circulation of red cells bearing mature stages of the parasite, (b) a peptide with a scrambled amino acid sequence was without effect, and (c) the *in vivo* and *in vitro* activity of HPLQKTY was strain transcending.

(3) Sera from individuals living in an area where falciparum malaria is endemic (and who are presumably immune) react with these synthetic peptides; such individuals are healthy i.e. not anemic.

(4) The critical amino acid residues in HPLQKTY that are necessary to block cytoadherence.

(5) The D form of HPLQKTY was as active as the L form, and the peptide YTKQLPH was as active as HPLQKTY.

(6) The mechanism for exposure of these peptidic regions is aggregation/ clustering of the intrinsic membrane protein of the red blood cell, band 3.

(7) Red blood cells treated with the oxidant t-butyl hydroperoxide expose the peptidic sequence YETFSKLIKIFQDH (also called the DIDS binding region, DBR), thus mimicking the changes in the malaria-infected red cell; moreover antibodies to the DBR (YETFSKLIKIFQDH) lysed such oxidant-treated red cells.

(8) Anti-DBR antibodies recognized band 3 aggregates (mostly dimers) from BS3 (bis-(sulfosuccinimidyl) suberate)-treated erythrocytes as well as from malaria-infected erythrocytes.

What is the significance of these findings? Development of *P. falciparum* within the red blood cell induces, in sequence, deposition of hemichromes and oxidative aggregation of band 3. This sequence of events is similar to that observed in normally senescent red blood cells or pathologic red blood cells, most notably sickle and thalassemic red cells. These membrane modifications of the red blood cell do not need primary involvement of parasite-specific proteins (but) the parasite is essential to provoke the membrane alterations. The exposure of cryptic amino acid residues of band 3 by parasitization and the immune responses to such may also serve to protect against severe malaria by preventing sequestration in those individuals who do not have sickle cell trait, glucose-6-phosphate dehydrogenase deficiency or β-thalassemia. The antibodies to HPLQKTY and YETFSKLIKIFQDH, and the peptides themselves, have the potential for preventing and treating falciparum malaria.

A physician in Florida (J. R. Kennedy) used the data accumulated by my laboratory to propose the development of a vaccine for malaria based on the augmentation of the immune response to regions of the band 3 protein that are cryptic in the uninfected red blood cell.[215] And, in a preliminary attempt at vaccination through the kindness of a colleague in Colombia (Socrates Herrera) a study was carried out in six *Aotus* monkeys to assess the safety, toxicity, and immune response associated to immunization with DBR synthetic peptide formulated in the adjuvants Freund and Montanide ISA 720. Monkeys were divided into three groups of two monkeys each: a control group, a Montanide ISA 720 group and a FCA group. Three doses of 100 μg were inoculated in the experimental animals on days 0, 20, and 40, with a boosting of 150 μg on day 60, because of low antibody titers. Control animals were inoculated intramuscularly using adjuvants without antigen in a similar schedule. Specific antibody titers against anti-DBR were determined by ELISA assays. All animals were challenged 85 days after last immunization with 1×10^5 *P. falciparum* FVO strain and parasitemia determined by thick and thin blood smears every day for one month. After four immunization doses with the DBR synthetic peptide on days 0, 20, 40, and 60, the monkeys developed low specific antibody titers as determined by ELISA assays. Follow-up carried out on days 0, 20, 40, 60, 90, 140, and 180 indicated that three animals developed positive anti-DBR antibodies that were more evident after the 3rd immunization. Inoculation of live parasites failed to produce a boost in antibody titer levels and complete protection was not observed, however, in a few of the Montanide animals there was a delay in the appearance of parasites in the blood. Importantly, antibodies to the DBR did not induce changes in hemoglobin or hematocrit levels.

Based on *in vitro* and *in vivo* studies I hypothesized: antibodies that specifically target the HPLQKTY and YETFSKLIKIFQDH, or the peptides themselves and/or derivatives of these, could be the basis for the development of synthetic non-peptide drugs and vaccines. However, neither USAID nor the NIH elected to fund further research into the possible use of the band 3 peptides or mimetics for vaccine development using monkey models.

The mainspring of my life as a malaria researcher has been a restless endeavor to get at the truth of things. Despite the vexations and frustrations of research there has been great delight, contentment and reward. I have been ambitious but not overly so. I have been competitive. Rivalry can drive innovation and absent competition there would be no need for publishing in peer-reviewed journals and no satisfaction in being the first to have an idea or a solution before anyone else. I have tried not to be over-confident and avoided over-interpreting our findings. My success in research, such as it has been, has taken diligence, perseverance, luck, and collaboration and throughout it has been hypothesis-driven.

In 2005, after more than 50 years of malaria research my extramural grant support terminated. By that time, the rivalry between researchers of PfEMP1 and pfalhesin/DBR had ended without there being a clear path to a protective vaccine. Trager had died, and Winograd returned to Colombia, Earlier, Ian Crandall had returned to Toronto. Most of the other graduate students and post-doctorals (Gruenberg, Allred, McDonald, Guthrie, Takahashi, Eda) who had worked with me left the field of malaria bio-chemistry/vaccinology. I closed down my laboratory, became an Emeritus Professor, and like a good soldier faded away.

Chapter 10

Vaccines to Halt Transmission

The oldest and most effective public health measures have been those interventions that prevented or reduced the transmission of malaria. In Italy in the early 19th century — years before Battista Grassi had implicated the mosquito in malaria transmission — legislation required that irrigated land be situated at least 500 m from rural habitations and at least 8 kilometer from towns.[2] In time, however, this approach toward reduction of contact between humans and mosquitoes by ensuring that the distance between the two was beyond the flight range of the breeding sites of the mosquitoes would be replaced by other methods designed to eliminate the mosquitoes themselves.

In April, 1899 Ronald Ross, then a Lecturer at the Liverpool School of Tropical Medicine, set sail for Sierra Leone. Sierra Leone, consisting of some satellite villages and its capital Freetown, was the British West African headquarters for trading and settlements on the Gold Coast. It was a black settlement firmly governed by whites and it prospered by trade with the interior. It was also disease ridden and remained the "White man's grave." The goal of Ross' project was to make Sierra Leone safe for white Europeans. By August Ross with his "army of mosquito extermination" identified the species of *Anopheles* that were the main transmitters; he then set about to eliminate the mosquito breeding sites. Ross' cheap and simple method i.e. draining the puddles where the mosquitoes bred, turned out to be a failure since the mosquitoes survived the dry season by using small pools in the stream beds and in the waste water and in spring runoff. In 1902, Sir Rickard Christophers and Captain Sydney Price James of the Indian Medical Service set out to eradicate malaria from a British troop contingent living in Lahore, India. The plan was simple: depress the mosquito population by clearing and oiling the irrigation ditches, removing infected individuals from the vicinity of the mosquito breeding grounds, and administering quinine to those who were infected. This too failed. The studies in Africa and India had proven that an attack on *Anopheles* was neither cheap nor easy, and mosquitoes were adaptable, and able to breed in a variety of water sources.

At the end of the 19th century the philanthropist John D. Rockefeller, funded a Foundation to wage war on malaria. In 1915, the Foundation announced it was "prepared to give aid in the eradication of this disease (malaria) in those areas where the infection is endemic and where conditions would seem to invite cooperation for its control." The Rockefeller Foundation employed over 400 scientists and sanitarians with a single-minded goal: eradicate malaria. Attempts at eradication were made by dusting with the insecticide Paris green (copper acetoarsenite) to kill the larvae of the mosquito. It worked, but only to a limited extent. By the beginning of the 20th century another transmission control was put into practice: eliminate adult mosquitoes by spraying with insecticides; initially pyrethrum powder and later dichloro-diphenyl-trichloroethane (DDT) were used. It was found that a single spraying of DDT to coat the interior wall where feeding mosquitoes rested halted the transmission of malaria for an entire season. Not only that it was simple and cheap. By 1945, the United Nations Relief and Rehabilitation Administration (UNRRA) decided on a campaign to eradicate malaria from Italy. It provided the DDT and money for the spray teams. In 1946, the Italian government took over the project and within three years the number of deaths due to malaria in Italy had been reduced to zero. The lesson learned in Italy was: DDT's value was not that it was more efficient than Paris green or pyrethrum in killing mosquitoes but that as a house spray it stood guard over an enemy that might recur in an area. It was a defensive weapon whose action resembled that of a vaccine.

DDT, by making the environment unsuitable for the transmission of the parasite, held out (for some) the possibility for the eradication of malaria. In 1947, the World Health Organization (WHO) was established and within it an expert committee on malaria. The committee's great hope was the eradication of the disease — and even *Anopheles* — from entire countries. Initially, they refrained from recommending an immediate worldwide campaign but by 1949 the experts at WHO had become impatient. An eradication campaign was sold to the nations of the world based on the near-miraculous blow that DDT dealt to malaria. In 1955, the World Health Assembly (WHA) endorsed an aggressive campaign to eradicate malaria by overwhelming force: interrupt transmission by insecticides and treat the infected people with antimalarial drugs. The WHO provided technical aid and UNICEF and United States Agency for International Development (USAID) provided the funding. In 1960, 52 nations that attempted eradication had a campaign completed or underway. Funding for the campaign peaked in 1965 and dwindled thereafter. By 1966, the WHA reviewed progress and noted that malaria had been eradicated from once endemic areas inhabited by more than 600 million people and had reduced the disease burden in another 334 million. Ten of the countries had achieved eradication, 11 others had banished the disease from some part of the territory. Of the 10 countries where eradication had been achieved four were in Europe, and the other 67 were in the Americas. Nevertheless, 638 million people still lived where malaria was actively transmitted and there it remained a major cause of morbidity and mortality. Not a single victory had been achieved in any major tropical area. There was a resurgence of malaria in places where malaria had been under control and the tide of disease had turned around. International organizations saw no end to the demands on their funds and with only diminishing returns from them became fed up. More and more the all-or-nothing WHO eradication campaign came to be regarded as a failure. An alternative to mosquito control by insecticides, and other sanitary measures, some have suggested, is to develop and deploy vaccines designed to limit the transmission of human malaria infections to mosquitoes — a transmission-blocking vaccine (TBV).

i. Mutualistic or Cooperative TBVs

A malaria TBV would not prevent disease in newly infected individuals, but would contribute to "herd immunity" in that, although it would not directly influence the course of infection in the vaccinated individual it would affect the potential for infection in others. Thus, TBVs are sometimes called altruistic vaccines. This, however, is misleading. Malaria is transmitted by mosquitoes over small distances, generally less, and often much less, than a kilometer. Indeed, a considerable amount of malaria transmission can occur between members of the same household. Thus, any measure that prevents an individual from infecting mosquitoes, such as a TBV, will significantly reduce the chance that others in a household will get malaria, and ultimately will reduce the chance that the vaccinated individual will be reinfected. In short, when it comes to malaria, as in other walks of life, what goes around comes around. Therefore, a house, a small community, a village, whose members elect to receive malaria TBV are not acting altruistically but are acting to their collective mutual and, indeed, individual personal benefit. Anti-mosquito stage malaria TBV is more correctly referred to as "mutually beneficial, or co-operative vaccination" (Carter, personal communication).

The path to a TBV began with Richard Carter (b. 1945). Late in 1967, after graduating with a B.Sc. degree in Biochemistry, Carter joined the Institute of Animal Genetics (which doubled as the Genetics Department of the University of Edinburgh) and the laboratory of Geoffrey Beale. Beale was one of the first to pick up upon the contributions that biochemical analysis, in the form of isoenzymes, could make to the investigation of genetic differences between organisms. Carter's task was to conduct starch gel electrophoresis analysis of "enzyme variation" in malaria parasites of rodents with the objective of obtaining "genetic markers" for use in crossing experiments between the parasites. These rodent malaria experiments were successful and after completing his Ph.D. Carter joined the NIH (National Institutes of Health) laboratory of Louis Miller.

In 1974, the talk of a "malaria vaccine" or "vaccines" was thick in the air at the NIH. Elsewhere, work was beginning on attempts to immunize against the blood stages of malaria parasites (see p. 74) to prevent or reduce the clinical effects of malaria, or to immunize against the sporozoites, and prevent infection altogether. What struck Carter, in the midst of this talk, was that unless either type of vaccine was 100% effective, neither would prevent malaria transmission in an endemic community. His experience as a malaria geneticist had already taught him that even a tiny number of gametocytes, such as might escape from "asexual" vaccination, and could very effectively infect mosquitoes. In Carter's mind, vaccination served one or both of two purposes, to reduce the risk of disease in a vaccinated individual, but equally, if not much more importantly, to reduce its spread to others.

None of these thoughts, however, were part of Carter's thinking until a day when there was a conversation that included himself, Miller and the NIH entomologist Robert Gwadz. Carter learned of Gwadz's interest in the possibility that infectivity of malaria parasites to mosquitoes could be modulated, in part, by host immunity. This was an idea first investigated more than two decades earlier by Don E. Eyles of the U.S. Public Health Service. Eyles had shown using the chicken malaria, *P. gallinaceum*, that serum associated with a peak in blood parasites was detrimental to the development of gametocytes in the mosquito.[216,217] Eyles had suspended gametocyte-carrying chicken red blood cells in a variety of chicken sera and fed these to mosquitoes through an artificial membrane. After a period of time Eyles carried out mosquito dissections and counted the number of oocysts on the stomach wall. Compared to sera from uninfected birds, that taken from chickens one day after the peak of a blood-induced infection caused a reduction in oocyst numbers indicating suppression of infectivity of the gametocytes to mosquitoes. As expected, normal chicken serum was without any effect on the number of oocysts.

Carter began to think more and more about the possibility of immunizing a host with the gametes of a malaria parasite (sexual forms which are normally to be found only in the mosquito midgut, but available now in the laboratory through the methods that he had been working upon). By immunization he mused, host antibodies against the surface antigens of the sexual forms would be induced. When ingested together with gametocytes in a mosquito blood meal, such antibodies would possibly do great harm to the gametes as soon as they had left the protective enclosure of the host red blood cell. The talk in the NIH laboratory was always about "anti-gametocyte" immunity and what might be going on in the host to harm the gametocytes as they circulated in the blood stream. There was no discussion, however, concerning the effects of an immunity that exerted its effects upon the gametes of the parasites as they were released into the mosquito midgut during a blood meal. At the time, the whole idea of antibodies, or other kinds of immunity of host origin, acting in the mosquito vector, tended to be disregarded, especially by professional immunologists, who more-or-less considered the notion to be non-sense. It was, therefore, with not a little trepidation, and a few days after the idea had occurred to him, that Carter put the concept, somewhat hesitantly, to Miller.

Carter remembers receiving a rather blank look — as happens when something almost ridiculously obvious has been put. But the implications in both their minds must have been jumping out at them. There was also the matter, and this was of concern to both Miller and Carter, that this was entering a research territory running very close to the interests being actively followed by Robert Gwadz. Although, neither Carter nor Gwadz had a stated goal at that point of working on anything directly to do with immunization for the purposes of suppressing infectivity of malaria parasites to mosquitoes, let alone making a vaccine, each was closing towards it from their own particular lines of investigation. What Carter proposed to Miller was the injection of extracellular gametes of *P. gallinaceum* into chickens to see whether there was any effect upon the infectivity of subsequent blood infections of *P. gallinaceum* to mosquitoes through the effects of antibodies on the gametes as they emerged into the blood meal.

Miller was supportive of the idea, but it was clear to both of them, that Carter would have to discuss it also with Gwadz and hopefully not find there was an unworkable conflict of interest. Carter went down the corridor to Gwadz's office and told him he was interested in testing the hypothesis that extracellular gametes of a malaria parasite could induce antibodies that would interact — not with the gametocytes in the blood stream of the chicken — but with the extracellular gametes in the mosquito midgut. This did not directly conflict with Gwadz's immediate research interest into the factors affecting infectivity to mosquitoes of *P. cynomolgi* infections in Rhesus monkeys. It did follow, however, from Carter's developing expertise in the preparation and handling of the extracellular gametes of malaria parasites. Thus in the spring, of 1975 the two agreed that Carter would conduct the experiments on gametes. As often happens in science, as in life, a plan, and the course of events do not always coincide. "Other things" intervened, delaying the start of Carter's proposed experiments by almost half a year — a set of experimental investigations had been already promised to a senior colleague in the UK. These now took precedence. And so, Carter left the NIH for a summer break at home in the UK where the idea for gamete immunization was discussed with Robert Killick-Kendrick, Robert Sinden, and the doyen of malaria, P. C. C. (Cyril) Garnham.

By the time Carter returned to the NIH that Fall he learned Gwadz had beaten him to the punch: he had immunized chickens with formalin-killed gametocytes of *P. gallinaceum*. Using a membrane feeding apparatus he showed that the gametocytes from the immunized chickens entirely recovered their infectivity when they were washed free of their own plasma and resuspended in normal chicken serum, whereas gametocytes from non-immunized chickens, when resuspended in serum from the immune chickens, were almost completely unable to infect mosquitoes. Then finally, he took the gametocyte-infected blood from the immune chickens and examined it under the microscope. There, for the first time, he observed the "microgamete immobilization reaction."[218]

The results were exactly — almost — what Carter had anticipated. What he had not envisioned was that this kind of immunity could have been induced by the gametocytes themselves, or at least not very effectively. This because part of Carter's thinking had been that such antibodies would be induced mainly by the stages that emerged in the mosquito midgut, i.e. by the gametes. He had anticipated that within the midgut of a blood-fed mosquito, a set of antigens would be expressed *de novo* on the gametes, and that these should be the targets of the immunity that would suppress their infectivity to the mosquitoes. In this way gamete vaccination would be a way of creeping up on the parasites unsuspected ... without any immune evasion mechanisms having been evolved.

After Gwadz's work there could be little doubt of the reality of anti-gamete infectivity suppressing immunity, essentially as Carter had thought.

Carter decided to go ahead with his original plans, in collaboration with David Chen, who had been hired earlier by Gwadz. They made semi-purified preparations of male and female gametes of *P. gallinaceum*, x-irradiated them to eliminate their infectivity to the chickens, and inoculated them directly, without adjuvant, into the chickens by the intravenous route. There were six such immunized chickens and one control. After three such weekly injections all the chickens were then infected with live blood stages of *P. gallinaceum*. Normal, or almost normal, blood infections ensued in all the immunized chickens and in the control. Mosquitoes were fed upon the chickens daily throughout their infections and the numbers of oocysts counted in the infected mosquitoes. The normal chicken produced the expected hundreds of oocysts throughout the infection. The immunized chickens produced either none at all at any time, or a very occasional one. The overall reduction in oocysts in the immunized chickens over the full course of their infections was 99.99–100% because the sera agglutinated and immobilized male gametes very effectively.

When Carter went to Gwadz's office and queried him about the successful immunization against the sexual stages of *P. gallinaceum* without any involvement on his part Gwadz rolled back in his chair and simply replied, "Ideas are cheap." Carter was taken aback, however, he would have been less so had he heard the words of the biochemist Nathan Kaplan: "good ideas are a dime a dozen for a smart person, and the only thing that alternately distinguishes good from great is in how an idea is executed — how it becomes reality." There is no reason to suppose that Gwadz and Carter had not approached their insights partially through their own independent thinking. They were certainly each traveling along apparently unconnected tracks that were, nevertheless, leading strongly towards the same destination. Yet without the other would either have taken the steps that led to the experiments that opened the field of malaria transmission-blocking immunity? Perhaps not, however, within the year Gwadz alone was awarded an NIH medal for the work.

ii. The Nature of Transmission-Blocking Immunity

After Carter began to explore more closely the mechanisms involved in anti-gamete immunity he coined the term "transmission-blocking immunity." The first study was an attempt to see whether extracellular gamete preparations were, in fact, any better than gametocytes. The results showed that exflagellated gametocytes did induce better transmission-blocking immunity than the exact same material that had been prevented from exflagellating before being used for immunization.

In the second study, using an *in vitro* system for fertilization developed from the experience from his experiments manipulating gametocytes and also using an ookinete culture system based on work by David Chen, Carter explored when and how the transmission-blocking antibodies exerted their effect. First, he investigated exactly when fertilization took place *in vitro*. When gametocyte-infected blood in glucose-saline, pH 7.4 was diluted 200-fold within 10 minutes, or sooner, after induction of exflagellation (male gamete formation), there was no subsequent formation of ookinetes (the products of gamete fertilization). However, when dilution was done more than 20 minutes after induction, the numbers of ookinetes that subsequently formed *in vitro* was the same as in never-diluted controls. Conclusion: fertilization must begin and be completed between 10 and 20 minutes after the induction of exflagellation. In a similar fashion, the transmission-blocking serum completely prevented subsequent ookinete formation if it was added before the moment of induction of exflagellation, but had no effect on subsequent ookinete formation when applied later than 20 minutes after the time of induction, i.e. when it was applied after fertilization had already taken place. In other words the antibodies were, indeed, fertilization-preventing antibodies.[219]

Carter went on to explore how, and for how long, the immunized chickens "remembered" the transmission-blocking immunity that had been induced by immunization with the gametes. It was found that up to at least six months after immunization and at a time when anti-gamete antibodies had ceased to be detectable in the circulation of an immunized chicken, a new blood infection dramatically boosted these antibodies back to effective transmission-blocking levels even before the first blood stage parasites were detectible in the blood. In short, the chickens' "remembered" almost instantly how to do transmission-blocking immunity as soon as they confronted a new malarial blood infection.

iii. Discovering the Antigens for a TBV

The next series of studies that Carter undertook with *P. gallinaceum* were devoted to characterizing the antigens on the surface of male and female gametes, and their developmental successors in the mosquito midgut, the ookinetes. The method involved using immune sera raised specifically against these parasite stages in chickens and rabbits, and monoclonal antibodies from gamete-immunized mice using the newly developed technology of Kohler and Milstein (see p. 126). Labeling the surface of gametes with radioactive iodine and then precipitating the now radioactive proteins using transmission-blocking monoclonal antibodies that reacted uniquely with either of these two specific protein antigens of the gametes identified two antigens. Such radioactive-labeled proteins were readily identified on a photographic film laid over a slab of gel in which they had been separated from each other by electrophoresis. As stated above, the monoclonal antibodies reacted with a single unique antigen, or actually a unique bit of an antigen called an "epitope," and thereby identified, as accurately as a DNA fingerprint, a specific protein. This and the fact that these particular monoclonal antibodies also efficiently blocked gamete fertilization and transmission of the parasites to mosquitoes, was proof that the antigens that they identified were the actual target antigens of the transmission-blocking immunity.

It was by these means, therefore, that the protein antigens that could be used for a malaria transmission-blocking vaccine were identified — at least for chicken malaria. The equivalent antigens of *Plasmodium falciparum*, were subsequently identified by the same methods.[220] These proteins of *P. falciparum* were named Pfs230 and Pfs48/45 based on their apparent molecular weight from migration through a gel under an electric field. These two antigens, Pfs230 and Pfs48/45, were expressed on the surface membrane of gametocytes as they developed inside the human bloodstream, and once the parasites were taken up in the blood meal by a mosquito they both remained associated with the surface of the emerged gamete for several hours. The anti-gamete activity of certain antibodies against these antigens, and especially against Pfs230, is dramatically effective.[221] When the antibodies are of the "complement-fixing" type they mediate their transmission-blocking activity by the lysis of male and female gametes and early zygotes within seconds to minutes; the destruction of these stages is effectively total. There are no survivors and no onward transmission of the parasites through the mosquitoes.

Meanwhile, still working with the *P. gallinaceum* system in chickens, Carter and his colleagues identified two additional antigens, Pgs25 and

Pgs28, on the developing zygotes of the parasites appearing respectively at around 5 and 12 hours after emergence.[222] Thereafter, the antigens continued to be present on the surface of the zygote throughout its development as an ookinete. Thus unlike Pfs230 and Pfs48/45, these antigens were expressed only during the mosquito phase of the malaria life cycle, and were not found at all in the gametocyte stages in the blood circulation. These proteins, too, were shown to be targets of very effective transmission-blocking antibodies. The mechanism of the effect of these antibodies remains unclear to this day. As had been the case with the gametocyte and gamete surface antigens, homologous protein antigens were then identified in *P. falciparum* and these were named Pfs28/Pfs25.[223]

iv. To Make a TBV

Plasmodium spp. have 14 chromosomes and the gene for Pfs230 has been located on chromosome 2. When the gene for Pfs230 is deleted the number of oocysts is reduced but not abolished.[221] At least one of the functions of Pfs230 is probably in fertilization itself, performing some essential action on the male gamete. It may also be that Pfs230 is involved in protection of the parasites from the digestive enzymes, nitric oxide, or against antimicrobial peptides within the mosquito blood meal. The gene for Pfs230 was originally cloned from a *P. falciparum* cDNA library. However, efforts to make a recombinant form of the Pfs230 protein that could be used as a vaccine have been difficult. These have largely to do with the fact that the protein is folded together by a large number of molecular bonds called "disulphide bonds." Disulphide bonds turn out to be extraordinarily difficult to reproduce accurately by synthetic means. So far only a small region of Pfs230 has been expressed in *E. coli* and to be able to induce antibodies with some transmission-blocking effect.[221]

Ps48/Ps45 is another identified target antigen of transmission-blocking antibodies that have their effect at and around the time of fertilization of the gametes of a malaria parasite in the mosquito midgut. Recently there has been a significant success in expressing Pfs48/45 in an immunogenic form that appears to have solved the riddle of how to recreate successfully the elusive disulphide bonds.[224]

One of the great potential strengths of Ps48/45 and Ps230 as antigens for a malaria TBV is that there can be a boosting effect. This was already anticipated in the Carter study on gamete immunization against *P. gallinaceum* in chickens[225] and subsequently in a powerful study with *P. knowlesi* in Rhesus monkeys.[226] This latter work showed that monkeys vaccinated with material containing gametes of a malaria parasite induced an immunity that had a very effective memory for transmission-blocking immunity of at least three years and no suggestion of it waning. At this point in time we do not know for how long such immune memory may last. It could be for so many years. If so, it would be of tremendous significance to the deployment of gametocyte/gamete antigen-based TBVs for the containment or even elimination of malaria transmission in endemic regions. Thus vaccinated populations could have their transmission-blocking antibodies boosted by incoming blood stage infections even many years after most malaria transmission had ceased, thereby locking out their onward transmission and sustaining a low malaria environment.

The likely reality of human immune memory for the gametocyte/gamete surface antigens has been shown in studies in malaria-endemic populations. Patients who experienced more than one *P. vivax* attack within four months had considerably less infectivity to mosquitoes than those experiencing their first attack suggesting the induction of transmission-blocking immunity by a prior infection. Moreover, antibodies to both Pfs230 and Pfs48/45 have been demonstrated in the sera of humans living in areas where *P. falciparum* is endemic area and the presence of these antibodies correlates with transmission-blocking activity in membrane feeding assays.[227,228]

In spite of the potential of the gamete surface antigens of the Ps230 and Ps48/45 type as TBVs, the most advanced of the TBV candidates are the post-fertilization antigens. Identification of the target antigens of anti-gamete immunity was pursued using monoclonal antibodies developed against purified *P. gallinaceum* ookinetes as immunogens. These monoclonal antibodies blocked transmission[229] and acted as would be expected i.e. well after the fertilization event. The effect was mediated by antibodies against a protein with a molecular mass of 26,000 (named Pg26) one of two *de novo* ookinete surface proteins — the other being a protein with molecular mass of 28,000.[230,231] These proteins are now known respectively as the Ps25 and Ps28 classes of ookinete antigens; they have been found in all species of malaria parasites investigated. The Pfs25 protein, the *P. falciparum* equivalent of the Pg26 ookinete protein, and Pfs48/45 has become the most advanced human malaria TBVs.

David C. Kaslow (b. 1958) grew up in Solvang, California and received a B.S. in biochemistry from the University of California, Davis (1979), and M.D. from University of California, San Francisco (1983). This was followed by a fellowship in human genetics in the Division of Pediatric Genetics at the Johns Hopkins School of Medicine. He joined the Laboratory of Parasitic Diseases at the NIH in 1986 where he worked on (among other things)[232] the identification and characterization of transmission-blocking antigens.[232–234] In 1986, a year after the transmission-blocking antigen Pfs25 was identified Kaslow set his sights on producing a recombinant protein. In 1988, Kaslow isolated the first gene encoding a target antigen of malaria transmission-blocking immunity, the one for the *P. falciparum* zygote/ookinete surface protein, Pfs25. The gene was isolated and sequenced by using degenerate nucleotides (based on the amino acid sequence of the three fragments) to screen genomic libraries. However, after failing to create a recombinant plasmid that encoded full-length Pfs25, he settled for a truncated version. Rabbits and mice vaccinated with the fusion protein produced an antiserum that recognized the native Pfs25, however, none blocked transmission. Undeterred, he made a recombinant antigen encoding the full-length Pfs25 using the WR strain of vaccinia virus, vSIDK, and produced an antiserum. Transmission-blocking antibodies recognized the surface of the vSIDK-infected cells expressing Pfs25, however, to produce potent transmission-blocking antibodies it took three vaccinations of mice. Although Kaslow had demonstrated a "proof of principle" that a TBV was possible by piggy-backing a malaria gene packaged in a virus, the project was abandoned because the virulent WR strain cannot be used in immune-compromised humans and some of the target population for malaria-TBVs have a high prevalence of HIV positivity.

Much of Kaslow's work with TBVs was done in collaboration with private industry. The success with the WR strain of vaccinia virus prompted an effort to develop an attenuated strain of recombinant vaccinia virus (NYVAC-Pf7). Although Pfs25 was expressed the antibodies produced did not reproducibly block infectivity to mosquitoes. Kaslow also pursued the expression of recombinant Pfs25 in yeast, bacculovirus-infected insect cells, and mammalian cells, however only in yeast were sufficient quantities of purified protein (Pfs25-B) made. Promising studies in primates using the adjuvant alum (suitable for use in humans) were not vigorously pursued after a mutual decision by the biotechnology company and the funding agencies to move the product to GMP production, and eventually further development of Pfs25-B was abandoned entirely. Redesign of the product, however, produced a new product, TBV25H, that was used in two clinical trials. In one, the Pfs25 was immunogenic but transmission-blocking activity was not observed. In a second trial the TBV25H was used to vaccinate human volunteers three times and was found to be immunogenic, however, because some of the volunteers had adverse reactions its safety remains to be determined.

In 1999, Kaslow left the NIH for Merck where he was senior director of vaccine research and then head of the Department of Vaccine Research and Technology; in 2001 he joined Vical Inc. In 2006, Kaslow returned to Merck as Vice President of the Division of Infectious Diseases serving as Vice President and head of vaccine project leadership and management at Merck Research Laboratories. In 2012, he joined the Program for Appropriate Technology in Health (PATH) as director of the Malaria Vaccine Initiative (MVI) to drive the development of safe and effective vaccines against malaria, and a year later PATH announced his appointment to the newly created position of Vice President of product development, effective October 1, 2013. In this new role he oversees the activities of all five of PATH's product development programs, as well as PATH's China programs, which also focus heavily on product development activities.

The recombinant form of Pfs25 has been evaluated in two phase 1 (safety) human trials.[234,235] A *Saccharomyces* expressed Pvs25 with allo-hydrogel as the adjuvant produced poor antibody titers with little transmission-blocking activity. When Pvs25 and Pfs25 were used with the adjuvant Montanide ISA there was some antibody response and transmission-blocking activity, however, the study was stopped when adverse reactions developed in the vaccines. A DNA construct encoding Ps25 was used to vaccinate mice and also produced potent antibodies capable of reducing oocyst numbers by 97% and decreased the number of infected mosquitoes by 75%, however to date no safety trials have been conducted in human volunteers.[236]

Preclinical studies have shown that *Pichia pastoris* produced Pfs25 when chemically conjugated to a detoxified *Pseudomonas aeruginosa* ExoProtein A (EPA) produces nanoparticles with an average diameter of 20 nm. When used with the adjuvant allohydrogel it resulted in higher titer antibody and transmission-blocking activity. A phase 1 clinical trial of this began in 2011 (ID Number NCT 01434381).[237]

Engineered virus-like particles comprising Pfs25 fused to Alfalfa mosaic virus (AMV) coat protein in the tobacco plant *Nicotiana benthamiane* were used to immunize mice with allohydrogel. Serum antibodies induced were able to block transmission for six months. A planned collaboration between the PATH MVI, the Fraunhofer USA Center for Molecular Biology, and Accelovance is to begin clinical development of this vaccine candidate.[238]

Although there is much promise in these novel approaches technical problems with the production of an effective TBV remain. In addition, even when successful production of a TBV is achieved significant challenges will occur in defining the development pathway where the endpoint is reduced transmission at the level of the community.

Chapter 11

Sporozoite Invasion
and the Path to RTS, S

By the early 1940s, with reports of the existence of protective antibodies in the blood of monkeys and birds (see p. 70) as well as the observation that the enhanced activity of serum used in treating *P. knowlesi* infections was directly correlated with the degree of "stimulation" of the immune system, there was a revival of interest in vaccination for malaria. Paul F. Russell and Major H. W. Mulligan at the Pasteur Institute of Southern India attempted to produce a protective vaccine using sporozoites. Believing that bird malaria was a reliable indicator for human malaria, Russell in collaboration with Mulligan used a simple sporozoite-clumping (agglutination) test to measure immunity in chickens infected with *P. gallinaceum*. When the chickens were in an acute or chronic state the agglutinin titer of serum was elevated. They then went a step further: when the salivary glands of mosquitoes heavily infected with *P. gallinaceum* sporozoites were placed in a shallow dish and exposed for 30 minutes to the direct rays of a mercury arc sun lamp the sporozoites were inactivated. Chickens vaccinated either intramuscularly or intravenously with these ultraviolet-irradiated sporozoites showed a considerable rise in the titer of sporozoite agglutinins. Further, of 14 chickens that received inactivated sporozoites and then challenged with viable sporozoites (by mosquito bite) 7% did not become infected, 64% recovered spontaneously, and 28% developed severe infections and died. Those suffering from the mild infection had a very high agglutination titer. They wrote "It seems fair to conclude, therefore, that repeated injections into fowls of inactivated sporozoites of *P. gallinaceum*, producing an agglutination titer of at least 1/32,000 render such fowls partially immune to the pathogenic effects of mosquito-borne infection with the homologous *Plasmodium*."[239] In another study they found that 92% of chickens with an agglutinin titer of 1/32,768 or higher showed spontaneous recovery and 8% died after challenge by the bite of infected mosquitoes whereas the mortality was 51% in chickens with normal or lower agglutination titers. Significantly, the immune chickens did not resist a challenge with intravenous injections of the same strain of blood stage parasites. They concluded: "this suggests that trophozoites and sporozoites are not immunologically identical."[239] In a subsequent report they noted the combined mortality for 19 fowls was 21.1%, which was less than half that of normal fowls similarly infected. This is a significant measure of immunization, although in no case was infection prevented.[239] Russell returned to the U.S. in 1942. During World War II, he served as a Colonel in the Army Medical Corps assigned to General Macarthur's headquarters in Australia. After the war Russell remained an administrator and technical advisor on malaria with the Rockefeller Foundation until he retired in 1959. In his classic work, *Man's Mastery of Malaria*, Russell provided a retrospective on the history of malaria and attempts at eradication, however, not a single sentence in the entire book refers to a malaria vaccine. Indeed, after his work in India and sporozoite vaccination, he never again was involved in trying to develop a malaria vaccine.

i. Vaccination with Irradiated Sporozoites

A group of investigators at the New York University (NYU) School of Medicine set out to determine whether *x*-irradiation of sporozoites might be a better source of antigen for vaccination than the ultraviolet-irradiated sporozoites that had been used by Russell, Mulligan, and Mohan. The NYU group was aware of the successful studies, carried out at the Walter Reed Army Institute of Research (WRAIR), using the *x*-irradiated infective larval stages (cercaria) of the blood fluke *Schistosoma* as a vaccine.[240] This vaccine not only prevented the worms from reaching the lungs and liver of the immunized host, there was a strong resistance to challenge. In most cases, the mean number of worms recovered from animals immunized with irradiated cercaria was 10% of the non-immunized controls. The percent reduction in the number of worms recovered was related to the number of immunizations up to the fifth immunization, with the duration of acquired immunity persisting for 119 days in mice, and 343 days in rhesus monkeys.[241] Success in the use of *x*-irradiation for reduction in the worm burden with blood flukes led quite naturally to vaccination trials with malaria parasites by the parasitologists/immunologists at NYU.

At the City College of New York (CCNY), Jerome Vanderberg (b. 1935), after taking courses in Ecology, Entomology, and Field Zoology with the most eminent lepidopterist in the United States, Alexander Klots, decided that he wanted to become an entomologist. However, a course in Parasitology (1954) convinced him that he wanted to work on things that had medical significance. Klots, like many of his generation, had spent World War II in the U.S. Army, in his case doing mosquito surveillance and control in the South Pacific. Therefore, Vanderberg worked in Klots' laboratory at the American Museum of Natural History on the mosquitoes that Klots had collected during the war. After receiving his B.S. degree (1955) from CCNY Vanderberg did graduate work at Penn State and then at Cornell and at the 1960 national meeting of the Entomological Society of America in Miami where he presented his Ph.D. thesis "The role of gonadotropic hormone in protein synthesis in *Rhodnius prolixus*" he wandered into a session on malaria and listened to a talk by Ian McGregor on the successful passive transfer of immunity by administration of immunoglobulin to children at risk. This work made it clear that vaccination against malaria might ultimately be carried out and convinced Vanderberg this was an area in which to work. Human malaria, however, does not lend itself easily, to basic research in immunology so a convenient laboratory model for *in vivo* studies of mammalian malaria was desirable. As often occurs with important discoveries, a Belgian physician (Ignace Vincke) and entomologist (Marcel Lips) were not searching for what they ultimately found. Vincke spent the years of World War II doing malaria surveys in the former Belgian Congo (now the Democratic Republic of the Congo). In 1942, he observed sporozoites in the salivary glands of the mosquito *Anopheles dureni*, collected near a major mining center,

Elisabethville (now Lubumbashi). Tests on the bloodmeal contents of the mosquitoes' midguts indicated the mosquitoes had fed on rodents or insectivores. When Vincke and Lips examined the blood of a local tree rat, *Thamnomys*, they discovered a new species of malaria, *Plasmodium berghei*. They postulated that the mosquito salivary gland infection with sporozoites observed years earlier and the newly described blood infection were due to the same species. Vincke named the parasite in honor of his close friend, Louis van den Berghe, of the Prince Leopold Institute of Tropical Medicine in Antwerp. However, it was not until 1950 that Vincke was able to show that sporozoites collected from these mosquitoes produced a typical *P. berghei* infection when injected into laboratory mice. Due to the graciousness of the Belgian workers, *P. berghei* was soon widely distributed throughout the world. Among the recipients of this rodent malaria parasite was Harry Most, who had worked on the development of chloroquine while in the U.S. Army during World War II and upon return to civilian life was Chairman of the Department of Preventive Medicine at the NYU Medical Center. During the 1960s most served as Chairman of the Armed Forces Epidemiological Board and Director of its Commission on Malaria, a civilian advisory panel. With the support of the Commission and funded by the U.S. Army Medical and Research Command a project on the biology of *P. berghei* was initiated at NYU.

Upon receipt of the Ph.D. (1961) Vanderberg worked as a postdoctoral fellow at Johns Hopkins University (1961–1963) studying mosquito physiology and transmission of *P. gallinaceum* in the laboratory of Lloyd Rozeboom. During a trip to New York City in May 1963, he learned that Most was interested in a medical entomologist, trained in insect physiology. He contacted Most, was interviewed, and before most advertised the position, was hired. Starting in September 1963, he immersed himself in what was known about the biology of *P. berghei* in Africa. During the next couple of years, his research was focused on working out the parameters for sporozoite transmission of *P. berghei* to laboratory rodents and the characterization of these infections in laboratory rodents. In 1965, the immunologist Ruth Nussenzweig joined the malaria research group (consisting of Most, Vanderberg and Meier Yoeli).

Immunization studies with *x*-irradiated rodent malaria sporozoites at NYU found the optimal dose of *x*-irradiation to inactivate the sporozoites dissected-out of mosquito salivary glands to be 8,000–10,000 rad; of 46 mice, each immunized via intravenous injection with 75,000 irradiated sporozoites, only one mouse developed an infection. The remaining mice were challenged 12–19 days later with 1,000 viable sporozoites.[242] The percentage of animals infected varied from 14–73% (average 37%) whereas in the controls the percentage of mice infected averaged ~90% and the protection was estimated to be 27–86%. There was no protection against an inoculum consisting of infected red blood cells confirming the stage specificity observed earlier by Russell and Mulligan. In a subsequent study of 103 mice injected with 75,000 sporozoites irradiated with 8,000 rad only three developed blood infections and with 10,000–15,000 rad none of 29 mice became infected. When the blood of the x-irradiated immunized animals was inoculated into other animals it failed to produce an infection and the immunized animals did not develop infections after removal of the spleen; this was taken to indicate that sterile immunity had been induced.[243] Protection remained strong for up to two months and then declined. By repeated intravenous challenge of immunized mice at monthly intervals, there was a boosting effect and protection could be maintained for up to 12 months.[244]

One of Vanderberg's most valuable finding was his observation that upon *in vitro* exposure to serum from immunized mice, an antibody-mediated precipitation reaction was formed around sporozoites, and projected from one end.[245] This reaction was called the circumsporozoite precipitation (CSP) reaction. The terminology for the CSP reaction was suggested by the similar appearing circumoval precipitation (COP) reaction around schistosome eggs incubated in immune serum. The abbreviation, CSP, originally referred to the CSP reaction however over time it has come, instead, to refer to the circumsporozoite protein. Because of the striking way in which serum from immune animals deformed sporozoites, this was postulated to be the basis for a humoral (= antibody) component of protective immunity against sporozoites. Indeed, incubation of sporozoites of *P. berghei* for 45 minutes with immune serum neutralized their infectivity. The CSP reaction was found to be produced in mice and rats immunized by intravenous inoculation with x-irradiated sporozoites of *P. berghei* or by the bite of infected x-irradiated mosquitoes, as well as in animals injected intravenously with viable *P. berghei* sporozoites.

Antibodies to CSP appeared to be critical to protection, however, because protection was never complete in passively immunized animals it suggested that additional mechanisms might be necessary to bring about complete protection against sporozoite induced malaria infections.

The discovery of the CSP reaction could have led to an enduring and productive collaboration between the members of the group at NYU, instead it created a rift, the basis of which had nothing to do with the findings *per se*, but with personalities and priority of authorship. Earlier, Vanderberg and Ruth Nussenzweig had an agreement that research publications on sporozoite "immunity" would have her as the senior author whereas those on sporozoite "biology" would have him as the lead author. Vanderberg, upon completion of his studies on the CSP reaction, prepared a draft manuscript. This was shown to Ruth Nussenzweig, who despite the fact that she had contributed nothing to the work directly, insisted on lead authorship claiming this was her research area. Vanderberg, on the other hand said the studies were conducted by him alone and concerned sporozoite gliding — a biological phenomenon. Most, as Department Chair, was asked to settle the conflict. He failed to support Nussenzweig's position, and as a consequence, a stressful and hostile environment was created. Henceforth, the members of the group were unable to work together in harmony.

With the initial success in the immunization of mice using x-irradiated sporozoites Ruth Nussenzweig recognized that it would be important to define the correlation between the *in vitro* detectable, anti-sporozoite antibodies, and protective immunity and to characterize the antigens involved. Emboldened by the results of the mouse vaccinations with x-irradiated sporozoites she assembled a team of immunologists to carry out investigations to isolate and characterize the antigens responsible for protection, and to extend the rodent malaria immunization studies to monkeys. Vaccination attempts were initiated using *P. cynomolgi* and *P. knowlesi* since in rhesus monkeys the former produces a mild and benign infection, similar to *P. vivax* in humans, whereas the latter is highly virulent and is more akin to *Plasmodium falciparum* infections in children. The results were disappointing: an initial study in two monkeys failed to protect against challenge after inoculation of x-irradiated *P. cynomolgi* sporozoites divided into five immunizing doses over a period of 146 days.[247] In a follow up experiment, using a dozen monkeys protection was obtained only after several months of intravenous inoculation of large doses of *x*-irradiated *P. cynomolgi* over a period of 9.5 and 13.5 months. However, only two of the animals were totally protected against challenge with 10,000–20,000 infective sporozoites.[246] With rhesus monkeys immunized multiple times with 300–400 million *x*-irradiated *P. knowlesi* sporozoites two monkeys developed sterile immunity, but not the third. There was no amplification of the anti-sporozoite protective response with *P. knowlesi* sporozoites emulsified with FCA administered intramuscularly nor was there protection against sporozoite challenge. Consequently, Ruth Nussenzweig abandoned, at least for the time being, further vaccination work on monkeys and directed her attention to characterizing the immune mechanisms seen with *x*-irradiated sporozoites in mice.

Vanderberg, in contrast to Ruth Nussenzweig, believed it was timely to carry out studies in humans. A collaborative arrangement was set up with David Clyde[247] at the University of Maryland School of Medicine where he was the director of a program studying anti-malarial drugs against sporozoite-induced malaria in human volunteers at the Maryland House of Correction in Jessup, MD. The irradiated sporozoite immunizations of human volunteers and subsequent challenge with un-irradiated sporozoites proved to be a long and sometimes frustrating effort because the first series of immunizations used X-ray doses that had previously been used with rodent malaria sporozoites. In those studies sporozoites had been directly obtained from dissected-out mosquito salivary glands, however, these could not ethically be injected intravenously into humans. An alternative approach was suggested from studies on mosquito-borne viruses. Serum surveys, done after epidemics of infections with these viruses, consistently showed that only a very small percentage of serum-positive individuals had actually experienced signs or symptoms of disease. Thus, from an epidemiological standpoint, mosquitoes might be more important as vehicles of immunization than as vectors of disease. The use of *Plasmodium*-infected mosquitoes to induce an infection was not entirely novel, its practice dating back at least to 1926 with the treatment of 2,500 patients with late-stage syphilis in England at the Horton Mental Hospital in Epson. (This treatment practiced in England, the U.S. and other countries persisted well into the 1950s, but with the widespread use of penicillin to treat syphilis, its usage declined.) The human trials first carried out by Clyde[248] and later by Rieckmann[249] would be a reapplication of this method for the purposes of testing the protective efficacy of a malaria vaccine.

Accordingly, an initial trial was conducted by Vanderberg with the rodent malaria, *P. berghei*, that used infected, *x*-irradiated mosquitoes as substitute "hypodermic syringes" to deliver sporozoites. The argument he made was: "the technique that we presently use for immunization involves the intravenous injection of infected mosquito salivary glands which have been dissected out, ground up and irradiated. However, this preparation contains considerably more extraneous mosquito debris than sporozoites, and the injection of such material into humans would possibly pose medical risks of embolisms and sensitization. Until sporozoite preparations can be purified it would seem prudent to avoid this. A more reasonable approach for the present would be to *x*-irradiate infected mosquitoes and then let them feed on volunteers, thus allowing the mosquitoes to inject the sporozoites in a relatively uncontaminated condition. Such a technique would have limited practicality, but it has the advantage of being performable now. If protective immunity could be demonstrated under such circumstances, it might encourage further work on attempts to establish purification procedures for sporozoite homogenates. The injection of irradiated sporozoites by mosquitoes should thus be viewed as an attempt to test the feasibility of vaccination in humans, which if successful could lead to trials using more practical techniques."[250] The results showed that mice so immunized were completely protected from sporozoite challenges that caused blood infections and death in 100% of non-immunized control mice. With the success of this approach, it seemed appropriate to move from mice to men.

The first series of immunizations of human volunteers used *x*-irradiated *P. falciparum* sporozoite infected mosquitoes. There were some breakthrough blood infections so several months were lost while retooling. A second series was begun with several new volunteers and with higher doses of *x*-radiation against the infected *Anopheles* mosquitoes.[248] An average of 222 mosquitoes that had been irradiated (17,500 rad) fed on each man and after 6–7 weeks each man was again fed on by an average of 157 irradiated mosquitoes. This time there were no breakthrough blood infections during the immunizations. The vaccinated individuals along with unvaccinated control volunteers were then challenged by bites of infected mosquitoes sufficient to have induced a blood infection in every single volunteer that had ever taken part in prior trials conducted by David Clyde and his associates. Upon challenge by the bite of mosquitoes infected with normal infectious sporozoites, one of three vaccinated volunteers was fully protected, whereas all of the non-vaccinated volunteers developed a blood infection, as expected. After the challenge, sporozoite-infected mosquitoes and serum from the challenged volunteers were brought to New York City. When Vanderberg tested these sera for reactivity with live sporozoites, strong CSP reactions were found in the serum of one of the vaccinated individuals (GZ). Vanderberg immediately telephoned Clyde and predicted that GZ would be protected. All were delighted when this prediction turned out to be true. It is perhaps relevant that GZ had taken part in the first vaccination trial, although he was not one of the vaccines who had experienced a breakthrough blood infection. Thus, he had received an especially extended schedule of vaccinations. They concluded that a sufficient dose of radiation-attenuated sporozoites was necessary to attain a sterile immunity upon challenge.

In 1974, Clyde began experiments on himself to determine whether it was possible to immunize against *P. vivax* as well as *P. falciparum* and whether there was cross protection.[251] Clyde allowed non-irradiated mosquitoes that were infected with vivax and falciparum malaria to bite him, and when he developed infections to both kinds of malaria he knew he was not immune. He described the first attack: "you shake like anything. You are very cold. You have a high temperature and a splitting headache. Then you start vomiting, and that is the most awful part of it. You have about four hours of absolute misery and then it gradually lets off for about another 12 hours. Then it starts again."[252] Clyde went on to see whether different strains had immunological differences and so he allowed irradiated mosquitoes from different geographical regions to bite him. Each time, he received scores of bites. "It was a damn nuisance and very unpleasant to have six cages of 350 mosquitoes hanging on to you but that's part of it."[252] The welts from the bites itched and he applied cortisone cream to relieve the irritation and to prevent himself from scratching. By the conclusion of the experiment he had received over 2,700 bites. To test the efficacy of the "vaccine" he accepted the challenge of being bitten by un-irradiated mosquitoes. He was protected. Unfortunately the protection was not long lived — in the case of falciparum three months and for vivax from 3 to 6 months.

Vaccination studies similar to those reported by Clyde, Vanderberg and Most, were conducted between 1971 and 1975 in a collaboration between the Naval Medical Research Institute and Rush-Presbyterian-St. Luke's Medical Center at the Stateville Correctional Center, Joliet IL under the direction of Karl Rieckmann.[249] Five volunteers were bitten by fewer than 200 *P. falciparum* infected mosquitoes x-irradiated with 12,000 rad over a period of 4–17 weeks and during the immunization two volunteers developed blood infections (which were quickly cured by chloroquine). This indicated the radiation dose was too low to inactivate all of the sporozoites. Of the four men challenged, none was protected. Another three volunteers were selected. One was exposed six times within a two-week interval; mosquito dissection showed that 440 mosquitoes had bitten him. Two weeks after the last immunization he was bitten by 13 infected non-irradiated mosquitoes and he did not become infected. A second volunteer was exposed eight times to a total of 984 x-irradiated mosquitoes and although the intervals were not exactly two weeks apart he too was protected against challenge 2–8 weeks after the last immunization; however, he showed no protection when challenged at 17 and 25 weeks after the last immunization. A third volunteer was exposed to 987 irradiated mosquitoes with immunization at irregular intervals during a 38-week period and when challenged eight weeks afterward with a strain different from that used in immunization was protected; however, when challenged with the same strain 18 weeks after the last immunization there was no protection. Thus, vaccination with x-irradiated sporozoites was "an encouraging step towards the goal of immunizing man against malaria" (Vanderberg, personal communication). The limited success of these vaccination studies served to establish what had been hoped for, namely, a clear "proof of concept," demonstrating that production of sterile immunity to malaria in humans might be biologically feasible and was deserving of further efforts.

ii. A Sporozoite Antigen Identified

Over 90% of adults living in The Gambia, an area of high malaria endemicity, were found to have detectable levels of anti-sporozoite antibodies.

Further, observations with rodent, human, and primate malarias showed that protective immunity mediated by immunization with x-irradiated sporozoites was associated with the induction of antibody. A monoclonal antibody raised against the surface of *P. berghei* sporozoites neutralized their infectivity,[246] and passive transfer with the monoclonal antibody protected mice against sporozoite challenge.[253] The sporozoite antigen of *P. berghei* recognized by the monoclonal antibody was stage and species specific, and was named the circumsporozoite protein, CSP.[246] Monoclonal antibodies were also prepared against sporozoites of *P. knowlesi* and *P. cynomolgi*; these were used to precipitate similar circumsporozoite (CS) proteins. As with *P. berghei*, sporozoite neutralization was associated with these monoclonal antibodies.

The CSPs from a variety of *Plasmodium spp.* are encoded by one gene (of the 5,300 malaria parasite genes). Ruth Nussenzweig, now joined by her husband Victor, was convinced that the CSP would be an attractive target for the development of a protective vaccine. Victor Nussenzweig (b. 1928) entered Medical School at the University of Sao Paulo in 1946 just after the end of World War II. Like many of his friends, he was impressed with the important role of the Soviet Union in the defeat of Nazi Germany, and was attracted to socialist ideals and Marxist ideology. During the first three years of Medical School, he was deeply involved in student politics. His future wife, Ruth, born in Austria and whose family emigrated to Brazil was in the same class, and when the two started dating she convinced Victor that science was much more interesting than politics. After receiving M.D. degrees Ruth and Victor went to Paris (1958–1960) with their two young children. Ruth worked at the College de France studying the metabolism of thyroid hormones, and Victor was accepted in the laboratory of Pierre Grabar at the Pasteur Institute working on antigen processing.

Back in Brazil Ruth and Victor worked with the prominent Brazilian immunologist, Otto Bier. In 1963, Victor received a Guggenheim Memorial Foundation Fellowship and came to the U.S. with Ruth and their three children, Michel, Andre, and Sonia. Ruth worked with Zoltan Ovary and Victor with Baruj Benacerraf at the NYU School of Medicine. It was an exciting time, a time when the structure of immunoglobulin was being solved. Although they tried to go back to Brazil in April of 1964, they were deterred because the military had just overthrown the elected government and started a witch-hunt at the University of Sao Paulo.

Therefore, they returned to New York City in October. In 1965, Ruth was appointed Assistant Professor in the Division of Parasitology at NYU where she began work on a sporozoite-based malaria vaccine. Victor, who had joined the Department of Pathology of NYU, and later would transfer to the Department of Preventive Medicine where Harry Most was Chair. Prior to Victor's transfer to the Department of Preventive Medicine. Most made overtures to the Pentagon that Victor, who was about to be deported back to Brazil for his prior socialist activities, remain in the U.S. since the Vietnam War was ongoing and therefore it was in the national interest for him to work on malaria. The entreaties worked. Victor was not deported and his career changed: he began work with Ruth on the Department of Defense funded rodent malaria project. The quest of Ruth and Victor for the "protective" antigen would lead, in succeeding years, to the cloning of the gene for the CSP, studies of CSP function in the initial stages of invasion of liver cells, the inhibitory role of gamma interferon (IFN-γ) in the development of the liver stages of malaria, and the demonstration that a CSP-based human vaccine against *P. falciparum* was possible.

In 1981, a practical impediment to the use of CSP as a vaccine was that its only source was the mature sporozoite. This difficulty was overcome by the cloning of the CS gene and the ability to deduce the amino acid sequence of the protein from the DNA base sequence. The first CS gene cloned was from *P. knowlesi*.[254] To clone the gene several thousand *Anopheles* mosquitoes were raised and fed on a monkey infected with *P. knowlesi* (done in collaboration with Robert Gwadz at NIH). At NYU the mosquitoes were hand dissected, the salivary glands separated and mRNA extracted from sporozoites by a graduate student (Joan Ellis) in the laboratory of the molecular biologist Nigel Godson. Three complementary DNA (cDNA) clones were obtained and the region that coded for the immunoreactive region was identified and sequenced. The cloning of the CS gene from *P. knowlesi* was quickly followed by the cloning of the CS genes from other human malarias i.e. *P. falciparum*, *P. vivax*, and *P. malariae* by several laboratories including those at the NIH and WRAIR.[255–258]

On February 12, 1981, NYU filed a patent application on behalf of the Nussenzweigs and Godson for their cloning of the CS gene. After filing the patent NYU notified the funding sources including USAID, NIH, and WHO and indicated that they were entering into negotiations with a genetic engineering company, Genentech, to produce CSP. When Genentech asked for exclusive licensing to market "the vaccine" objections were raised by WHO which indicated that their support required "public access" and under U.S. patent law USAID held the patent for the work it supported at NYU. The conflict dissipated in 1983 when the NYU-based research had moved ahead accomplishing the work that was to be done by Genentech. The bargaining over the market rights were discouraging to the Nussenzweigs who were falsely accused among other things of having a financial stake in the patent. The legal wrangling however continued for years. In the end it was resolved and the achievement by the NYU group was heralded in an August 13, 1984 NY Times headline "Malaria vaccine is near."[259] One scientist quoted in the article boldly predicted: "this is the last major hurdle. There is no question now that we will have a vaccine. The rest is fine tuning." In 1989, NYU licensed the CSP patent non-exclusively to GlaxoSmithKline (GSK), royalty free; this ultimately would lead to the malaria vaccine RTS, S (see below).

The gene sequences of all CSPs code for 300–400 amino acids, with the central region consisting of tandem repeats of amino acids rich in the amino acids asparagine (N) and proline (P) separated by the amino acid alanine (A) and flanked by two regions of highly conserved amino acid sequences, designated region I and region II. (The region II has been suggested to be involved in the sporozoite binding to and invasion of liver cells.) The CSP of *P. falciparum* has six repeats and is often written as $(NANP)_6$. Screening a large number of sporozoites from different areas of the world showed that all isolates had the same repeats although variations occurred at other regions of the CSP.

When human volunteers were given three intramuscular injections of a conjugate of tetanus toxoid and $(NANP)_3$ in alum there was a good correlation of the antibody titers of anti-peptide and anti-sporozoite antibodies. However, when three of the individuals with the highest titers were challenged by the bites of five heavily infected mosquitoes, two had a prolonged period (i.e. 11 days vs. 7 days) before parasites appeared in the blood and only one individual did not develop a blood infection.[260]

In another study under the auspices of WRAIR, volunteers were given (again via the intramuscular route) a recombinant NANP protein (R32NS181) formulated with a more potent adjuvant (MPL, monophosphoryl lipid A, a cell wall skeleton of mycobacteria and squalene). Six of the 11 volunteers had high CSP titers; two of these did not develop an infection when bitten by five *P. falciparum*-infected mosquitoes and two had a delay in the appearance of blood parasites.[261] WRAIR also conducted a trial of a recombinant protein produced in *E. coli* consisting of 32 NANP repeats and 32 non-relevant amino acids. When used to immunize 15 individuals, 12 developed antibodies to the NANP repeats but the titers were low (1:500 and 1:1,000). Six of those immunized were challenged with sporozoites; in the volunteer with the highest antibody titer no parasites were found in the blood and in the other two the appearance of blood parasites was delayed.[262]

Although the work with human volunteers suggested that a CSP based subunit vaccine might be feasible, it was clear that "not everyone with high titers of antibodies to the repeats was protected, however, those who were protected had high antibody titers."[263] In addition, it was evident from the NANP-tetanus toxoid vaccine study that although the antibody response was dose dependent there was a limitation: the levels of the carrier protein, tetanus toxoid, could not be increased, as they were toxic.

iii. WRAIR and RTS, S

In the 1960s, the appearance of chloroquine resistance by *P. falciparum* in Southeast Asia and South America provoked a renewed interest in controlling the mortality and morbidity from malaria: indeed, at the beginning of the Vietnam War (1959–1975) the number of U.S. soldiers evacuated from wounds inflicted by enemy forces was equal to that from malaria. The need to protect and treat U.S. forces led the U.S. Congress to expand funding for research into malaria, and in 1963, the U.S. Army Research Program on Malaria was launched at WRAIR. Most of this was devoted to a search for new antimalarials and by 1974, 26 new drugs or combinations had been developed, 11 clinical trials were completed, with mefloquine being the flagship response to chloroquine-resistant *P. falciparum*, however, a substantial proportion was allocated to basic research, including immunology.

In 1963, Elvio Sadun (1918–1974), Chief of Medical Zoology of WRAIR and Special Assistant to the Director for Basic Research in Malaria was asked to explore new approaches to current problems with malaria.[264] Sadun was born in Livorno, Italy and because of virulent anti-Semitism under Benito Mussolini was forced to emigrate to the U.S. in 1939.[265] He received an M.S. degree at Harvard under L. R. Cleveland (who was also the major professor for William Trager), served in the U.S. Army in North Africa and Italy and then completed a Ph.D. at the Johns Hopkins University studying immunity in chickens to the roundworm *Ascardia galli*. In 1951, Sadun accepted a commission in the U.S. Public Health Service and was assigned by the USAID to Thailand where he conducted surveys on worm infections. Returning to the U.S., he was appointed Head of Helminthology at the CDC where he evaluated new antigens and developed serological tests for trichinosis and hydatid disease. Following a two-year stint in Japan, he was appointed (in 1959) Chief of Medical Zoology at WRAIR a position he held until his death in 1974. Although a "worm immunologist" by inclination and training Sadun recognized that one of the unfortunate consequences of the illusion that insecticides and drugs could eradicate malaria was a decline in biological research; he also noted that DDT went further toward the eradication of malariologists than it did mosquitoes. Consequently, Sadun organized a program at WRAIR to conduct basic research in malaria, to attract highly capable scientists from various disciplines to carry out malaria research, and to produce a continuing flow of highly trained people able to contribute to the management and control of this disease.

One of those who joined WRAIR to study the immunology of malaria was Carter Diggs. Carter Diggs (b. 1934) grew up in sight of the Piankatank River, which empties into the Western side of the Chesapeake Bay where he saw (and ate) a lot of marine biological specimens. Using a primitive microscope he saw for the first time paramecia in water collected from jars of standing water. Truly awed, he became a microbe hunter. As an undergraduate (Randolph–Macon College in Ashland, VA), and still on the trail of microbes, he declared himself a biology major and since most of his colleagues majoring in biology were headed for medical school, he followed the path of least resistance and applied too!

Graduating from Randolph-Macon College (June 1956) he enrolled at the Medical College of Virginia (MCV) in the fall and soon found he did not want to practice clinical medicine, but instead wanted to do some kind research. His first experience in a research laboratory was with Robert Marston where he worked on isolation of viruses from children with aseptic meningitis and found that most cases that summer in Richmond were due to Coxsackie B-5. (Marston would go on to become director of NIH.) During the summer of his junior year at MCV he worked on several projects, but the one that sticks out in his memory was the (accidental) discovery of a serum trypsin inhibitor; a very exciting moment until he found out that it had been discovered some decades earlier! These experiences reinforced the idea that he wanted to be involved in research and so he applied for an internship and residency in pathology at MCV.

The year following receipt of the M.D. he worked in the morgue doing autopsies and in the pathology laboratory reading slides from tissues. The experience was valuable but he knew he didn't want to spend a career at it. During the second year of pathology, Diggs received a letter, which began: "greetings from the President of the United States." It directed him to show up at a certain date for induction into the U.S. Army, but included a note at the bottom indicating that since he held an M.D. degree, he did not have to show up on that date if he had applied for a commission before then. His boss, George Margolis, knew some people at the WRAIR and an appointment was set up. As a result, he obtained a position in the Division of Communicable Diseases and Immunology (DCD&I) directed by Colonel Abram S. Benenson.

After basic training at Fort Sam Houston, Carter showed up at WRAIR early in 1962, reported to Benenson, and discovered there was a Department of Immunochemistry in DCD&I headed by Elmer Becker. Becker's area of research was complement, however, the word around was that Becker might have an interest in the function of the lymphocyte, a subject about which essentially nothing was known. Diggs had been looking at lymphocytes infiltrating sites of chronic diseases during the year in the pathology laboratory and this provoked a keen interest in what in the world they were for. When Benenson asked Diggs what he'd like to do, he immediately told him he'd like to work with Becker on lymphocyte function. He said he was sorry but there were no slots available in that laboratory and suggested visiting all the labs in DCD&I and then come back to talk some more about an assignment. After visiting the Departments of Virology, Rickettsiology, Bacteriology, Medical Zoology, Applied Immunology, Molecular Biology, and Serology as well as Immunochemistry Diggs told Benenson he was still interested to work with Becker on the lymphocyte. Benenson said he was very sorry but there was no slot there, but there was one in Medical Zoology and he needed someone to start thinking about vaccination against malaria.

The next week Diggs reported to Sadun in Medical Zoology. Sadun was under pressure to pay attention to malaria. He instigated a meeting to kick off the malaria effort ("Cultivation of Plasmodium and Immunology of Malaria") and supported Diggs in his fledging efforts at malaria immunology. At the time, Diggs was the only one in the department working on malaria! The first thing Diggs did was to get some *P. berghei* from NIH where there was some work going on (albeit nothing in malaria immunology, he remembers). A considerable amount of Diggs' time during 1962–1964 was devoted to trying to isolate parasites, immunizing rabbits with the crude parasite extract and doing electrophoresis and immune precipitation to try to identify malarial proteins. He got lots of lines of precipitate (= precipitins), but didn't progress much beyond that.

By this time, convinced that he needed more training in immunology he applied to the Army for a Ph.D. program, at the Johns Hopkins School of Medicine and in due course, was approved and moved to Baltimore in time for courses in the fall of 1964. His mentor at Hopkins was Abraham Osler, a very bright, knowledgable, and meticulous immunologist specializing in allergy. Although not engaged in malaria research, Osler was a great humanitarian and Diggs' desire to learn how to engage in malaria vaccine development tweaked his interest from that point of view. In addition, Osler's own training was under Michael Heidelberger, who unsuccessfully attempted to produce a vaccine from lysed infected cells (see p. 73).

Leaving Hopkins, Diggs was assigned directly to the SEATO laboratory (now the Armed Forces Institute of Medical Sciences) in Bangkok, Thailand to head the Department of Parasitology. During the two years there (aside from administrative chores) he introduced some serologic techniques and supported the ongoing fieldwork that had been started by others. In 1970, he returned to WRAIR and the Department of Medical

Zoology where he had the pleasure of working with Bruce Wellde. Bruce came to WRAIR in uniform as a corpsman and quickly developed into an independent scientist. With Wellde, Diggs studied aspects of immunization against malaria with irradiated parasitized erythrocytes,[266] a little celebrated phenomenon and at about the same time the group at NYU showed protection induced by x-irradiated sporozoites. They also demonstrated a delayed appearance of parasites in the blood of *Aotus* monkeys passively administered IgG from Nigerian donors at the time of infection with blood stage *P. falciparum*.[267]

In 1973, a number of events converged to change the administrative structure at WRAIR. As WRAIR moved more and more to the applied research and development, the Department of Immunochemistry was judged to be too focused on basic research to be justified. Another Department, Serology, was phasing out as personnel retired. At about the same time, Sadun developed hepatocellular carcinoma from which he succumbed. The upshot of it all was that a new Department Immunology, was formed out of the three and Diggs was appointed as Head.

In time, malaria vaccine development became the sole mission of the Department of Immunology at WRAIR. In 1975, in collaboration with a young physician, David Haynes, *P. falciparum* was cultured for 10 days. The key to their success was gassing the cultures with CO_2. Haynes had done cell culture at Yale University and was sensitized to the CO_2 requirement in a number of systems as a component of the buffer system in the medium. He had approached the problem very systematically and appreciated the anaerobic nature of malaria parasites. As often happens in science, Haynes *et al.*[268] were not the only ones who cultured *P. falciparum* that year. Trager and Jensen published before them. This was the scoop of a lifetime and while the Trager–Jensen discovery was celebrated (see p. 65), the Haynes–Diggs culture system was forgotten.

After Diggs made a site visit to the laboratory of Miodrag Ristic to consider Department of Defense funding of ongoing USAID-supported malaria vaccine work at the University of Illinois using "exoantigens" as the basis of vaccines, it was discovered that the "exoantigens" were a "gemisch" and efforts to correlate protection with a component in it were not promising. The Ristic project was not recommended for funding, however, now Diggs entertained the idea of looking at the gemisch to see whether it contained any interesting antigens. At the time, a senior fellow from France, Daniel Camus, had come to work at WRAIR and Diggs asked him to look at what was in the spent *P. falciparum* culture medium using immune serum. Together with a young investigator, Terrence Hadley (who had been in the Army, worked at WRAIR and was making a transition to NIH to work with Louis Miller) the two had other ideas: what was in the spent medium that would stick to red cells? The experiment involved exposing fresh uninfected red blood cells to the spent culture medium, washing the cells and determining whether the immune serum agglutinated the red blood cells. It did, and thus a new antigen was discovered: erythrocyte binding antigen or EBA-175.[105]

In 1979, Franklin Top vacated the Directorship the DCD&I to become WRAIR Deputy Director and Diggs was asked to fill the slot while continuing as Chief of Immunology. One of his first jobs was to pick a successor to head up Immunology. The choice was obvious: a young officer, Wayne Hockmeyer, who had just finished a tour as Director of the WRAIR unit in Nairobi. Keen to develop an immunoassay for detection of falciparum sporozoites in mosquitoes Diggs contacted Ruth Nussenzweig's laboratory, which had just published on the development of monoclonal antibodies against CSP, and, with those, he reasoned it would be a snap to develop such an assay. The only problem was Ruth had the monoclonal antibodies and wouldn't part with them. When asked for the monoclonals or the hybridoma cell line, she assured WRAIR they could have them ... but not just yet. She wanted to be sure her students had time to submit their papers. Or, there was too little supply right now. Or, there was some other problem, and this went on for about a year. At that point, the group at WRAIR decided to make their own monoclonal antibody, not a trivial task in those days. With effort and an excellent team, WRAIR soon had its own CSP monoclonal antibodies.

By this time, the group at NYU had identified the CS gene for *P. knowlesi*. Diggs recognized that this might allow for a well-characterized antigen for vaccine development and so the decision was made at WRAIR to go all out to develop a falciparum vaccine using recombinant DNA methods. However, at the time WRAIR had no molecular biology capacity, but it did have a monoclonal antibody! Then, Diggs got a got a call from Louis Miller of NIAID who said they had developed a *P. falciparum* genomic library and proposed: probe the cDNA library with the WRAIR monoclonal antibody to look for the CS gene. The arrangement, to which Miller agreed, was to be a full collaboration and WRAIR would have access to any materials that came out of the shared work. Haynes took the initiative to be the main WRAIR hands-on collaborator, working with John Dame and Tom McCutchan at NIAID. Within a week, plaques of bacteria were producing CSP.

Once CSP was available, the work on a vaccine took off thanks to a very active collaboration between GSK and WRAIR and in which Wayne Hockmeyer took the lead for WRAIR. The vaccine (named FSV-1) was developed in record time, being much less hampered by regulatory constraints than is the case now. Hockmeyer (who was a Ph.D. not an M.D.) arranged for infectious disease fellows in training at Walter Reed Hospital to do their research elective in the department, thus building a clinical vaccine testing capacity. The subjects were primarily the staff, and all but one subject who received the vaccine developed malaria on challenge.[262] Although the trial was considered a failure, in retrospect, that one subject who did not become infected was an important lead. He had the highest antibody titer, was repeatedly challenged and still he didn't become infected (although he finally did). The protected volunteer wasn't Diggs ... although he had a chill the night before becoming slide positive feeling only a little tired before the chloroquine took effect whereas others were extremely sick!

Not long after the initial vaccine trial, and now more than five years beyond the obligatory 20 years in the U.S. Army, Diggs had reached the pinnacle at WRAIR (with the title of Associate Director for Plans and Overseas Operations) and he began to search for the next career move. It was at this time that the USAID Malaria Vaccine and Immunology Research (MIVR) Program had run into serious trouble (see p. 89), and it seemed here was an opportunity to make a greater contribution to malaria vaccine development than by his staying at WRAIR. Phillip Russell, Commanding General of the U.S. Army Medical Research and Development Command, and a former colleague at WRAIR, had the ability to assign Diggs to USAID while still on active duty.

The first year (1988) at USAID was stressful for Diggs. At that time, health activities were under the Bureau for Science and Technology, and, it appeared that there was open warfare with the rest of the Agency! Some at USAID believed the entire malaria vaccine development effort should be abandoned. In addition, there was a GAO audit of the program going on as well as an investigation by the Inspector General (see p. 89).

When Diggs took the helm of the MIVR, most people were looking at the first clinical trial of an NYU peptide-based vaccine as a failure, although there was significant delay in the onset of the appearance of parasites in the blood. The results of the trial, along with the scandal at USAID, made for a painful period. In a manner similar to the loss of enthusiasm for malaria eradication 20 years earlier, there was much pessimism regarding the feasibility of ever developing a malaria vaccine.

Diggs' mandate at USAID was to reorganize and reorder the priorities of the MIVR as well as to trim the program to fit the reduced budget. Continuing support of the University of Maryland Center for Vaccine Development (CVD) was seen as not cost effective since clinical trials were not envisioned for the next several years. Similarly, the development of a field trial capability in Papua New Guinea (PNG) was not going to be used for vaccine trials in the near future. USAID funding for both was terminated. Fortunately, the CVD had multiple streams of income and survived this without too much difficulty. The PNG operation was stressed more severely, but muddled through, and the facility USAID built was put to good use. A similar fate was met by the USAID funded malaria laboratory at the Biomedical Research Institute in Rockville, MD as well as most of the rest of the old portfolio. Under the "healing process" the program underwent, all investigator initiated research projects were subject to periodic external peer review, and none survived more than a few years. At present Diggs is the Senior Technical Advisor to the USAID Malaria Vaccine Development Program and he continues to work towards the development of malaria vaccines to protect children and other vulnerable people in endemic areas.

iv. RTS, S

The decade's long quest to develop a safe and effective subunit malaria vaccine is instructive in delineating the hurdles faced in the production and testing of a vaccine, the critical importance of having good collaborations, and the empiric nature of vaccine development. In early 1984, after the scientists at WRAIR had cloned and sequenced the *P. falciparum* CS gene it became possible to develop a subunit vaccine. WRAIR entered into collaboration with GSK to produce CSP using GSK's recombinant *E. coli* expression system. Although efforts to produce a full-length CSP were unsuccessful, four constructs were expressed, purified, tested for immunogencity in animals and one (R32Ltet32) was selected for clinical development. Combined with alum (as an adjuvant) the vaccine, FSV-1, was tested on volunteers in 1987.[262]

Ripley Ballou, then a young U.S. Army physician and five colleagues (including Stephen Hoffman from NMRI, see p. 106) taped a mesh-covered cup containing five infected anopheles mosquitoes to their arms. The *Anopheles* were allowed to bite them and afterward, to make certain the mosquitoes in the cup were infective, the heads of the mosquitoes were lopped off in Ronald Ross-like fashion using a pair of tweezers and the salivary glands examined with a microscope. Ballou and the other volunteers had been injected a year earlier with FSV-1 and now it was time to be challenged with infectious sporozoites to assess protection. Nine days after the infected mosquitoes had fed the first unvaccinated control had parasites in his blood and was given chloroquine to clear the infection. The second control and three vaccinated volunteers also came down with blood infections and on the 11th day Hoffman, confident the vaccine would work and had traveled to San Diego to give a presentation on the vaccine, fell ill with malaria. On the 12th day, Ballou also succumbed. Only the sixth volunteer Daniel Gordon was still healthy and remained so. The efficacy of the vaccine was disappointing, however, for the first time an individual had been completely protected by a subunit vaccine. When the vaccine was tested by WRAIR for safety and immunogenicity in western Kenya the majority of vaccinated subjects had antibodies to CSP.

Over the next several years, a series of recombination constructs of CSP (R32NS1$_{81}$V20, R32NS1$_{81}$) were produced by GSK that incorporated the NS1$_{81}$ protein from the influenza virus to stimulate helper T lymphocytes; when these were tested with volunteers at WRAIR the immunogenicity of R32NS1$_{81}$V20 was low and further clinical development was not pursued. In parallel, WRAIR tested R32NS1$_{81}$ in combination with the only acceptable adjuvant for use in humans, alum (called

FSV-2) and although it was more immunogenic this too failed to protect any of the volunteers. FSV-2 in combination with other adjuvants including MPL, or an emulsion of MPL, mycobacterial cell wall skeleton and squalene (Detox, Ribi Immunochem), and cholera toxin were also tested at WRAIR but again the results were disappointing.[269]

In 1990, Gray Heppner volunteered for a vaccine trial at WRAIR. Heppner who was raised in Lynchburg, VA did his undergraduate work at the University of Virginia and after completing his M.D. at the University of Virginia Medical School did an internship and residency at the University of Minnesota where in the late 1980s he had assisted a malaria researcher growing *P. falciparum* and in the process became intrigued with malaria. Although Heppner joined the Army Reserves while in Minnesota, he didn't sign on for active duty until 1990 and that brought him to WRAIR as an infectious disease officer. At WRAIR the CSP lacking a central repeat region, called RLF had been expressed in *E. coli* and when encapsulated in liposomes was found to be immunogenic in mice; further the anti-RLF serum reacted with the surface of intact sporozoites and was able to inhibit their invasion into liver cells *in vitro*. The safety and immunogenicity of the RLF vaccine was tested in 17 malaria-naïve volunteers, Heppner being one of them. Although RLF formulated with alum or MPL was well tolerated and immunogenic upon sporozoite challenge all immunized volunteers developed malaria.[270]

In 1987, the GSK malaria vaccine program transferred its labs in Philadelphia, PA to its vaccine division in Rixensart, Belgium. Joe Cohen, who had taken over the project at the same time that Ballou and colleagues at WRAIR had been using themselves as human guinea pigs, had another plan for using CSP as an antigen. Cohen, using experience gained from GSK's successful development of a recombinant hepatitis B vaccine, Engerix-B, decided to couple CSP with the surface antigen protein from hepatitis grown in yeast (*Saccharomyces cerevesiae*) where at high concentrations the protein spontaneously formed virus like particles, and when used as an immunogen antibody formation was enhanced. Cohen hoped that by fusing the NANP repeat from CSP to the hepatitis surface antigen (consisting of 226 amino acids) similar particles now festooned with the active epitope of CSP would be made and be able to provoke antibodies targeted to the sporozoite surface. To overcome the possibility that antibodies alone would not suffice Cohen added a fragment from the tail end of CSP to stimulate T cell responses. This construct would provide, as Cohen said, a "double whammy" with 19 NANP CSP repeats (R), T cell epitopes (T) fused to the hepatitis B surface antigens (S) co-expressed, and self-assembled with unfused S antigen. It was named RTS, S.[269,271] In 1992, the first clinical trial of RTS, S for safety and efficacy was carried out at WRAIR using volunteers. Malaria-naive volunteers received RTS, S either with alum or alum plus MPL. Both formulations were well tolerated and immunogenic, however, after challenge with sporozoites zero out of six in the alum group and only two out of eight in the alum-MPL group were protected. Significantly, one protected subject had an increased T cell activity against CSP.[272] These results were considered to be encouraging enough to warrant further improvement in the vaccine to enhance both humoral and cell-mediated immunity.[273] Taking clues from the study, Heppner cooked up a formulation with adjuvants that would produce the right sorts of cell-mediated immune responses. Heppner suggested formulating RTS, S with an oil in water emulsion plus the immunostimulants MPL and QS21 (a proprietary GSK saponin derivative from the Chilean soap bark tree, *Quillaja saponaria* (AS02), and by 1996 — 12 years after the first trials — RTS, S/AS02 was tested in human volunteers and protected six out of seven vaccines. When the volunteers were challenged six months later one of five volunteers was still protected. Two or three intramuscular inoculations were necessary to produce sterile or partial immunity (i.e. delayed appearance of parasites in the blood) in most vaccines. In liquid form the RTS, S/AS02 had a limited shelf life and so the RTS, S was freeze-dried and then reconstituted with AS02. When 40 volunteers received the vaccine on a 0, 1, and 3-month schedule or on a 0, 7, 28-day schedule of vaccinations protection against sporozoite challenge was seen in 45% and 38% of the vaccines, respectively.[274]

In the summer of 1998, trials were held in The Gambia with 250 men receiving RTS, S/AS02 or a rabies vaccine on a 0, 1, and 3-month vaccination schedule. The RTS, S showed a 34% reduction in the first appearance of parasites in the blood over a 16-week period. During the surveillance period 81 of 131 men immunized with RTS, S had parasites in the blood whereas in the control group 80 out of 119 tested positive. The following summer the men were given a booster and this showed that the vaccine was acting in two ways: protecting against infection and weakening the symptoms in those who became infected.[275]

Although GSK was encouraged, the company felt it needed funding assistance to move RTS, S into trials with infants[276] Ballou wrote a proposal to the Bill and Melinda Gates Foundation and it provided $50 million through the Malaria Vaccine Initiative (MVI) through the Program for Appropriate Technology in Health (PATH). Ballou was asked to lead it, but instead took a position with a Washington, DC biotechnology firm, MedImmune, to work on other vaccines. In 1999, Heppner succeeded Ballou as Chief of the WRAIR Malaria Program, and in 2006 becoming Director of WRAIR's Division of Malaria Vaccine Development. Retiring in 2011, he has held positions at Crucell Inc. (2011–2012), TASC (2012–2015) and is currently Chief Medical Officer of BioProtection Systems/New Link Genetics Corp.

With the MVI on board GSK and WRAIR collaborated with Pedro Alonso of the Barcelona Center for International Health in Spain who had developed a research site in Mozambique. Alonso's site would be the biggest RTS, S trial enrolling 2,022 children between the ages of 1–4 years. By 2003, Ballou had rejoined the effort having left MedImmune to join GSK at Rixensart. The trials in Mozambique with children showed that the vaccine conferred a 35% efficacy against the appearance of parasites in the blood and a 49% efficacy against severe malaria that was maintained for 18 months after the last vaccination. Another formulation specific for children (RTS, S/AS02D) was tested in 214 infants in Mozambique in preparation for licensing. Infants were given three doses of RTS, S/ASO2D or the hepatitis B vaccine Engerix-B at ages 10 weeks, 14 weeks, and 18 weeks.[276] Early on, 17 children in each group had adverse reactions and later 31 had serious adverse reactions none of which seemed to be related to vaccination. Vaccine efficacy for new infections was 65% over three-month follow-up after completion of immunizations. The prevalence of infection in the RTS, S group was lower than in controls (5% vs. 8%). The reason why 35% of the children did not respond was not clear nor why the vaccine protected only 34% of adults and was of shorter duration. Perhaps it stems from problems associated with induction of immunological memory.

In a collaboration between GSK, MVI and 13 clinical centers in eight sub-Saharan countries an RTS, S phase 3 study begun in 2009, involved two age groups of African children: 5–17 months and 6–12 weeks at the time of enrollment (RTS, S Clinical Partnership, 2011). The children were vaccinated with RTS, S/ ASO1, co-administered with diphtheria-tetanus-pertussis-hepatitis B-*Hemophilus influenza* type B pentavalent vaccine and a Sabin polio vaccine. After one year in the 5–17 month old children there was a 55.8% reduction in the incidence of the first or only episode of clinical malaria and a 47.3% reduction in the incidence of severe malaria. In the 6–12 week old infants, 14 months after the first dose of vaccine, the reduction in the first or only episode of clinical malaria was 30.1% and the efficacy for severe malaria was 26%. After four years vaccine efficacy was 16.8%.[277] In July 2014, GSK applied for regulatory approval of RTS, S for use in African children.

It has been suggested that both humoral and cell-mediated immunity contribute to protection with the RTS, S vaccine with the relative importance depending on the pre-existing immune status of the individual and as yet other undetermined host factors. The reason why antibody alone does not eliminate incoming sporozoites is not understood, however, it may be that continuous shedding of CSP-antibody complexes allows the highly motile sporozoites to escape. RTS, S vaccination may reduce but not completely prevent emergence of the merozoites from the liver, so that vaccinated children receive an attenuated low level blood infection that allows a more effective immune response to the asexual (and disease causing) blood stages.[278]

Questions remain: how long will the RTS, S vaccine protect? Will efficacy vary according to the intensity of transmission? How often will individuals need to be re-vaccinated in order to stop all the parasites from appearing in the blood to cause disease? And, how much will the vaccine cost?

Chapter 12

Attenuated Plasmodial Vaccines

i. X-Irradiated Sporozoites of *Plasmodium falciparum*, PfSPZ

Since the 1980s subunit malaria vaccines have received the most attention and it is sobering to note there is only a single recombinant protein vaccine on the market for any disease, and no vaccines based on synthetic peptides, recombinant viruses, recombinant bacteria or DNA plasmids. In stark contrast, protective studies with *x*-irradiated sporozoites of rodent and human malarias have fared better than subunit vaccine formulations. In 1989, *x*-irradiated sporozoite immunization studies were begun at Naval Medical Research Institute (NMRI) and Walter Reed Army Institute of Research (WRAIR) using volunteers.[279,280] After 10 years of clinical experience with these immunizations Luke and Hoffman concluded: "immunization with radiation-attenuated *P. falciparum* sporozoites provides sterile protective immunity in >94% of immunized individuals for at least 10.5 months against multiple isolates of *P. falciparum* from throughout the world."[281] They went on to write: "given the ... need for an effective ... malaria vaccine ... we believe that an attenuated sporozoite vaccine should be produced and tested for safety and protective efficacy as soon as possible." And, echoing the words of Paul Silverman (see p. 81) that the hurdles associated with a whole parasite vaccine were simply technical problems that could be overcome by a major, well-funded research program, Hoffman wrote that "although technically and

215

scientifically challenging such an approach has an enormous advantage over other approaches." Shortly thereafter, (2002), Hoffman founded and became the CEO of the only company in the world dedicated solely to developing a radiation attenuated sporozoite vaccine for malaria. The name of the company Sanaria — meaning, "Healthy air" is a clever counterpoint to the Italian word malaria, namely "bad air." In 2005, Hoffman filed a patent (200050220822) for "aseptic, live, attenuated sporozoites as an immunologic inoculum" and began the difficult task of putting theory into practice.

Stephen L. Hoffman (b. 1948), currently the Chief Executive and Scientific Officer of Sanaria, was heralded in the December 11, 2007 NY Times as "the soul of a new vaccine." Impatient and intolerant of negativity he is following the century-old precepts of Louis Pasteur to turn a crippled malaria parasite into a wonderful protective weapon against itself. By 2001, Hoffman had to come to the conclusion that it would take many more years to develop a highly effective malaria vaccine based on recombinant DNA technology. He retired from the Navy and joined Celera Genomics as Senior Vice President of Biologics with the goal of utilizing genomics and proteomics to produce new biopharmaceuticals, especially immunotherapeutics against cancer. While at Celera he organized a Keystone Symposium on malaria vaccine development, and left the meeting frustrated by the realization that biotechnology was unlikely to produce a highly effective malaria vaccine for at least another 25 years. However, in putting together data from 10 years of work immunizing people with radiation-attenuated sporozoites he came to the conclusion that already there was a way to make a malaria vaccine. The approach had been pioneered decades earlier by the group at the New York University (NYU) Medical Center (Nussenzweig and Vanderberg) using rodents and later tested with human volunteers in Maryland and Illinois (Clyde and Rieckmann). Believing this approach would provide a highly protective malaria vaccine, he left Celera in 2002 and founded Sanaria in his kitchen with a single goal in mind: develop a malaria vaccine for infants, young children, and women using a disarmed version of the whole malaria parasite. Malariologists had always considered radiation-attenuated sporozoites as the "proof of principle" that a malaria vaccine could be developed, but none thought that a vaccine composed of radiation-attenuated sporozoites that met regulatory and cost of goods requirements could be manufactured. The accomplishments made by Sanaria during the succeeding years have shown an *x*-irradiated sporozoite vaccine can be manufactured. Clinical lots have been produced, and the vaccine, called PfSPZ, has now been shown to be safe in pre-clinical animal studies.

Hoffman is not a newcomer to malaria vaccines. Indeed, in the Spring of 1987 as a Commander in the Navy Hoffman was part of a team of military physicians involved in the test of a circumsporozoite protein (CSP) based subunit vaccine and at that time was so confident in the vaccine (FSV-1) he allowed himself to be bitten by 3,000 infected mosquitoes and then 10 days later went off to a medical conference in San Diego, California to deliver what he thought would be a triumphant message. The morning after he landed, however, he was already shaking and feverish, and shortly thereafter he was suffering with a full-blown attack of falciparum malaria. Clearly, the subunit vaccine was a failure, and Hoffman concluded that vaccination using a single malaria protein would never do the job of achieving full protection against the complex malaria parasite with more than 5,000 proteins.

Hoffman's approach has been to develop a whole sporozoite vaccine. Initially, he obtained $15 million in backing from the U.S. Army, a San Francisco non-profit pharmaceutical company, Institute for One World Health, and another $29 million from the Bill and Melinda Gates Foundation to allow the building of an assembly line of workers to mass produce the vaccine. This involves raising mosquitoes aseptically, supercharging them with far more parasites than nature does by membrane feeding the mosquitoes on blood containing *in vitro* grown gametocytes, allowing two weeks for the sporozoites to mature in the mosquito salivary glands, *x*-irradiating the infected mosquitoes, and finally dissecting out the sporozoites from salivary glands. It has been claimed by Hoffman that four trained dissectors working in two biosafety hoods can aseptically isolate sporozoites from at least 75 mosquitoes per dissector; this he believes would be enough for 1,200 three-dose immunization regimens. With two shifts per day and 310 workdays a year a small factory with 50 full-time dissectors per shift could produce 110 million doses of vaccine per year. These *x*-irradiated sporozoites would then be placed in suspended animation in liquid nitrogen until needed for immunizing human volunteers.

In 2010, the first clinical trial of the vaccine, PfSPZ, was conducted in humans who received up to six doses of 135,000 *x*-irradiated sporozoites administered either subcutaneously or intradermally. The vaccine was well-tolerated however only two were protected against challenge while all the other volunteers (vaccinated or unvaccinated) developed blood stage infections in 11–15 days after challenge. Hoffman hypothesized that the limited efficacy was due to the route of administration, and therefore it might be necessary to administer the vaccine in other ways to increase its effectiveness.[282]

Undeterred Hoffman's group teamed up with Robert Seder of the Vaccine Research Center (VCR) at the National Institute of Allergy and Infectious Diseases to immunize three Rhesus monkeys with the PfSPZ vaccine. The results showed that the intravenous rather than the subcutaneous route 'elicited potent and durable PfSPZ-specific T cell responses in … blood and most notably in the liver, the likely site of immune protection."[283] Rhesus monkeys cannot be infected with *P. falciparum*, but when the vaccine was used in a mouse model they found the level of protection was 71–100% using intravenous administration. The difference from injection into the skin was 'staggering' Hoffman said. "It was an aha moment," added Seder.[283] Following this finding in mice, they were emboldened to conduct a phase 1 clinical trial to determine safety, immunogenicity, and protective efficacy with intravenous immunization in human volunteers. In 2012, the PfSPZ vaccine — composed of radiation attenuated, aseptic, purified, cryopreserved sporozoites — was administered four to six times intravenously to 40 adult human volunteers; none of six subjects receiving five doses over 20 weeks, and three of nine subjects receiving four doses developed malaria when bitten by infected mosquitoes. The results of the study were published in the September 20, 2013 issue of *Science* (and publicized in the August 8, 2013 of *Nature News* with the headline "Zapped malaria parasite raises vaccine hopes" (http://www.nature.com/news/zapped-malaria-parasite-raises-vaccine-hopes-1.13536). In August 12, 2013, a *NY Times* article had a more cautious (and realistic) headline: "a malaria vaccine works, with limits." "Although these results are encouraging many challenges remain before this vaccine might be licensed for widespread use … and it required more than 600,000 sporozoites per subject to induce complete immunity."[284]

The Sanaria vaccine is slated for a trial at the Ifakara Health Institute in Tanzania, and Hoffman hopes to have the vaccine licensed in four years. When Hoffman was questioned about the vaccine being a scientific advance rather than a practical one he responded: "our goal has always been to show that this vaccine is highly protective. Once we have done that we'll figure out how to make it practical."[285] Despite his claims the Sanaria vaccine is impractical for malaria-endemic countries for the following reasons: the vaccine is made in small batches by hand, has to be stored in liquid nitrogen, and giving multiple doses intravenously is also tricky. Further, this vaccine requires sterile conditions, well trained medical personnel, and it will be difficult giving it to small children whose veins are hard to find. It is also unclear how long protection lasts, what the costs of PfSPZ will be, and whether it will work against all strains of *P. falciparum*. Although Seder calls the results 'very promising' he cautions that the study sample was quite small. "We need to repeat it in a large number of people" noting that in a 1997 publication of a trial of RTS, S the vaccine protected six out of seven adults in one group yet that level of protection was never achieved in subsequent trials.[285]

ii. Mind the Genetically Attenuated Parasites (GAPs)

Other laboratories have been working on vaccines similar to PfSPZ, however, instead of using radiation-attenuated sporozoites, they are using GAPs as a component of a protective vaccine. Indeed, the availability of genome sequences, the generation of stage-specific gene expression data and the ability to genetically manipulate the malaria parasite have enabled investigators to search for those genes that are essential for parasite survival. The most successful use of GAPs has come indirectly from studies that were designed to identify the virulence genes of sporozoites needed for successful transmission.

Stefan Kappe (b. 1965) always had a strong interest in Biology, majoring in it during high school and spending many happy days collec-ting beetles in the woods around the German town, Bad Homburg, where he grew up. Subsequently he received a diploma thesis (Master equivalent in Parasitology (1991) at the Rheinische Friedrich-Wilhems University in Bonn, Germany, working on host cell invasion by two relatives of malaria parasites (*Eimeria* and *Sarcocystis*). In 1992, he joined John Adams laboratory at the University of Notre Dame where he studied molecular events in red blood cell invasion using rodent models. Upon completion of the Ph.D. (1998) he applied for an advertised position in the laboratory of Victor Nussenzweig at the NYU Medical Center. At the time, the Nussenzweig laboratory was focused on CSP but in collaboration with Robert Menard the group had recently used reverse genetics to analyze the function of thrombospondin related antigenic protein (TRAP). Kappe studied the role of TRAP in sporozoite gliding and invasion. The group at NYU was exceptional as a breeding ground for new ideas and great projects. Although it was obvious that there had to be other interesting molecules in sporozoite biology in addition to CSP and TRAP no one knew how to identify these. So Kappe took up the challenge and made the first high quality cDNA library of *P. yoelii* salivary gland sporozoites. He remembers telling Steve Hoffman about having succeeded, and hearing his response: "impossible." In collaboration with Kai Matuschewski (now at the University of Heidelberg) Kappe used suppression subtractive cDNA hybridization and found 30 distinct genes in salivary gland sporozoites that were upregulated, and of these 29 were not significantly expressed in blood stage parasites.[286] These genes were called "up-regulated in infectious sporozoites (UIS)." Using the rodent malaria *P. berghei* it was possible to attenuate sporozoites by deletion of UISs. The genes for UIS3 and UIS4 encode proteins of the parasitophorous vacuolar membrane found in liver stage parasites and when these were deleted there was complete arrest of EE development after sporozoite invasion of the liver. However, the UIS4 'knockout' showed occasional breakthrough blood infections when high numbers of infectious sporozoites were used for vaccination. Deletion of two other sporozoite-expressed genes: P52 which encodes a GPI-anchored protein and P36 encoding a putative secretory protein, also aborted EE development in the liver, but these also yielded breakthrough blood infections. However, when both P52 and P36 were deleted there was complete attenuation and no appearance of blood stage parasites. (Recall that all of the pathology of malaria is due to parasites reproducing in the blood). Immunization of mice and with all four genes deleted in sporozoites induced long-lasting protection against a subsequent challenge with infectious sporozoites. These GAPs induced protection mainly by the production of CD8 T lymphocytes but antibody itself also contributed.[287] Deletion of sporozoite asparagine-rich protein1 (SAP1) also resulted in the arrest of EE stages in the liver and mice immunized three times with 10,000 of these sporozoite GAPs were protected against challenge with infectious sporozoites for at least 210 days.[288] Interestingly, it was subcutaneous inoculations of the sporozoite GAPs, not intravenous inoculation that yielded the best protection against challenge. In 2002, the Seattle Biomedical Research Institute offered Kappe a position in their fledging malaria research program. Feeling it important to leave the NYU 'nest' and start a truly independent program he moved to Seattle in 2003. In 2004, Kappe, Matuschewski, and Mueller filed patents 7,261,884 and 7,122,179 and an international patent application PCT/US2004 for a "Live Genetically Attenuated Malaria Vaccine."

The Kappe laboratory is currently engaged in the systematic identification of liver stage-expressed proteins and so far has identified ~800 proteins. In collaboration with other laboratories, Kappe is evaluating new antigens as targets for cellular responses using immune cells taken from animals that have been immunized with the live-attenuated sporozoites.

Kappe and coworkers have identified equivalent GAPs in *P. falciparum* and created the first gene deletion strains of Pf52/Pf36 double gene knockouts in collaboration with Alan Cowman's group at WEHI. In 2013 Kappe and coworkers carried out the first human proof-of-concept safety and immunogenicity clinical trial of GAPs in six human volunteers. Vaccinations consisted of Pf52/Pf36 deleted GAP *P. falciparum* sporozoites delivered via *Anopheles* mosquito bite with a five bite/volunteer exposure followed by an ~200-bite/volunteer one month later.[289] Three weeks following exposure to five bites, all volunteers were negative for blood parasites. Five of the six volunteers remained negative after exposure to ~200 bites; the one individual not protected developed parasites in the blood 12 days after the high dose (~2,000 bite) exposure. The findings indicated that attenuation had been incomplete in the Pf52f/Pf36 deleted GAP.

Since deletion of two sporozoite genes was less than optimal a trial was conducted with a triple gene deletion, by knocking out the SAP1 gene shown to be essential for EE development in the mouse malaria, *P. yoelii*. Using *P. falciparum* this triple gene-deleted GAP (PfGAP) was indistinguishable from wild type parasites in blood and mosquito development and when a sporozoite challenge was used in a humanized mouse model (having human liver and human blood cells) this 'next generation GAP' did not transition to a blood stage infection and was completely attenuated.[289] This, the authors suggest, warrants clinical testing for safety, immunogenicity, and efficacy against sporozoite challenge in human volunteers. In a subsequent study[290] immunization with the PfGAP vaccine resulted in a strong antibody response and plasma collected three months after the last exposure to the vaccine inhibited sporozoite invasion.

In the future optimization of genetic attenuation and determination of dosage will be critical before there is a safe protective GAP-based vaccine, however, even when this is achieved the most formidable obstacles for the GAP vaccine approach will be the need for production of sufficient numbers of viable, aseptic sporozoites as well as for cryopreservation in liquid nitrogen.

iii. A Live Blood Stage Vaccine?

The pioneering work of Edward Jenner with smallpox and Louis Pasteur with rabies demonstrated that dead or attenuated pathogens are able to act as effective vaccines. Indeed, whole organism vaccines, both live-attenuated and killed represent 75% of presently licensed formulations for bacterial and viral infections including polio, rabies, cholera, influenza, whooping cough, typhoid, plague, diphtheria, and attests to their safety and efficacy. For malaria however whole parasite vaccines have been viewed as impractical due to the complexity of the parasite's life cycle as well as logistical and safety concerns relating to manufacture. Ever since the classic failure of Heidelberger (see p. 73) to protect against infection using killed asexual stages of *P. vivax* there has been a tendency to shy away from the use of whole blood stage parasites. As a consequence, even with the possibility of producing large amounts of *P. falciparum* infected red cells in the laboratory using Trager–Jensen cultures, the last 30 years has seen most of the effort devoted to developing subunit vaccines (recombinant, synthetic or genes-based constructs) that would protect through immunization. However, since such strategies have not yet proved very successful there has been a resurgence of interest in immunization using radiation-attenuated or genetically attenuated sporozoites (see p. 219) and blood stage parasites followed by treatment with antimalarials. In the latter case a strong cellular immunity was induced that led to a delay in the appearance of parasites in the blood. Following this lead Michael Good[290] proposed and tested a strategy for vaccination using blood stages.

In a preliminary study naïve human volunteers were given four ultra-low doses of 30 *P. falciparum*-infected red cells at five-week intervals, followed by drug cure (with atovaquone-proguanil) 6–8 days later, and after the fourth challenge they were given chloroquine on day 14.[291] (With this regimen there were four rounds of parasite multiplication and no clinical symptoms were observed). After challenge there was a strong immune response characterized by a proliferation of CD4 and CD8 T-lymphocytes and IFN-γ production in the absence of antibody. Three of the four volunteers were fully protected. It was suggested (but not proven) that the immunity was cross-reactive.

Good and coworkers extended these studies using a rodent (*P. chabaudi*) model by treating infected red cells with irreversible DNA alkylating agent sec-cyclopropyl pyrrolo indole analogs that block parasite replication. After vaccine administration, without adjuvant, parasite DNA was detected in the blood for 110 days at fluctuating levels suggesting that active replication was occurring albeit at a very low level. The replication of parasites appeared to be limited since transfer of blood from vaccinated mice into naive recipients did not produce a blood infection. A single immunization induced strain transcendent immunity. Vaccine efficacy required the presence of intact red blood cell membranes and the antigens expressed during the ring stage appeared to be responsible for a protective immunity that was not antibody based.[290,292]

Before vaccination of humans with a chemically attenuated parasite is to be attempted there are major issues to be addressed. What are the hazards involved in the administration of a blood product for prophylaxis that could contain other blood-borne pathogens to many thousands of healthy individuals? The fact that the chemically altered malaria parasites did multiply in the body suggests that this could result in significant pathology including anemia and fever; and such a 'vaccine' consisting of infected blood may select incoming parasites that are antigenically variant. Still unresolved is whether the immunity attained was actually sterile, whether immunized individuals would remain protected against a subsequent infection with a higher dose of parasites, and whether there would be protection against sporozoite challenge. And a critical question is: will the rodent model using *P. chabaudi* translate into an efficacious multispecies vaccine for humans?

History has shown that the protective vaccines most easily developed against bacteria and viruses have been those that induce natural immunity after a single infection. For falciparum malaria the situation is different: clinical immunity develops only after several years of exposure to malaria-infected mosquitoes. This is generally assumed to be the result of parasite antigenic variation, as well as the ability of the malaria parasite to interfere with the development of an immune response. Vaccine strategies that are likely to be successful for protection against malaria are those that combine many antigens to induce a maximal response to a protective determinant that might not normally be recognized after infection of immunologically naïve individuals. Some have suggested that an alternative to multivalent vaccines would be to use attenuated parasites or ultra-low doses of whole parasites. However, as already noted there remain significant obstacles to these "back to the future" approaches. In the end, the greatest value in a whole organism malaria vaccine may be that it will allow for the identification of those target antigens that are critical to protection, something not yet achieved.

Chapter 13

Viruses and Plasmodial Vaccines

In the early 1990s the main focus of the vaccine program at Naval Medical Research Institute (NMRI) led by Stephen Hoffman was on DNA vaccines with special emphasis on EE stages and immunity to these in the liver. Indeed, when the program was started, DNA vaccines seemed to overcome the impediments of more traditional recombinant protein subunit vaccines. DNA-based vaccines induce both CD8 T lymphocyte responses (to produce the interleukin IL-12 and gamma interferon (IFN-γ)) as well as T helper lymphocyte responses (to release the interleukins IL-4, IL-5, IL-6, and IL-10); these are simple to design and modify, can be combined easily, are stable, do not require refrigeration and can be produced on a large scale. In 1993 a plasmid DNA encoding a portion of the circumsporozoite protein (CSP) from *P. yoelii* was used to immunize mice[293]; as predicted from experience with other systems the levels of CD8 T lymphocytes and IFN-γ increased. A year later when mice were immunized with a plasmid encoding another yoelii antigen and were protected against sporozoite challenge, it encouraged the development of DNA-based vaccines for use in humans. Indeed, the combination of DNA plasmids was pursued by the NMRI in partnership with Vical Inc. in a program called Multistage DNA Vaccine Operation (MuStDO).[294] The initial clinical trial in human volunteers tested the efficacy of a five plasmid mixture of pre-blood (sporozoite and EE) antigens (CSP, thrombospondin related antigenic protein (TRAP), LSA-1, LSA-3, and Exp-1). As with the mouse malaria DNA vaccine antigen-specific CD8 T lymphocytes and IFN-γ responses were found in the human volunteers. The vaccine was safe and well tolerated when given at four-week intervals. Subsequent studies varied the effectiveness of the route of vaccination. "However, despite the induction of cytotoxic T lymphocytes (CTL) and IFN-γ responses by each of three different routes of DNA administration ... in the frequency and magnitude of the responses was suboptimal and probably not adequate for protection ... Antibodies were not detected in humans by any of the different routes of DNA administration despite the same DNA vaccine having been shown to induce antibody responses in mice, rabbits, and monkeys."[295] Even in mice strain differences in response were observed and in those where there was protection it did not withstand challenge doses and protection was short-lived. Further, although the vaccine did provide evidence for priming in that the immune responses were boosted in the vaccines after being exposed to sporozoite challenge there was no protection.[296]

Such disappointments using plasmid DNA vaccines led to another approach: using virus vectors. Viruses, when modified, have the advantage of being able to serve as vaccine carriers being able to deliver DNA more efficiently than in the form of plasmids, however, they may have a drawback in that they might divert the immune response to irrelevant virus antigens and possibly neutralize pre-existing antibody responses to viral components. The NMRI vaccinologists elected to take advantage of both plasmid DNA and viruses by using a complex regimen: a priming dose of plasmid DNA and boosting with a recombinant virus. An initial trial with *P. knowlesi* and rhesus monkeys used a cytokine-enhanced multi-antigen DNA plasmid encoding two sporozoite antigens (CSP and TRAP) plus two blood stage antigens (apical membrane antigen 1 (AMA-1) and merozoite surface protein, (MSP)-1$_{42}$) for priming, and a canary pox virus was used as a booster. Two out of 11 rhesus monkeys (18%) vaccinated showed sterile protection and seven out of nine (77%) vaccinated rhesus monkeys spontaneously recovered.[297] In a subsequent and more detailed study with priming by three doses of DNA plasmids containing a mix of the same four *P. knowlesi* antigens and then boosting with the pox virus it was concluded: 1. The timing of vaccination and formulation were critical to protective efficacy, 2. Protection could be achieved in some animals against both pre-blood and blood stage infections, and 3. In a multistage vaccine the individual antigens may interfere with one another. A perplexing finding of these experiments was that although the vaccine was protective the IFN-γ responses correlated with an earlier appearance of parasites in the blood.[298] Clearly another approach was needed.

The viruses that cause the common cold and other respiratory diseases, belonging to the group named adenovirus (Ad), have found utility as gene vectors. Ad vectors induce both humoral (antibody) and cell-mediated responses simultaneously and can protect after a single immunization. Most Ad-based vaccine vectors contain a single foreign gene, however, it has been possible to generate Ad vectors that can carry several genes and express multiple proteins. Currently, the U.S. Military Malaria Vaccine Program, and the University of Oxford are developing Ad vectors able to carry several falciparum proteins in the hope that this array will serve as the basis of an effective protective vaccine.[299]

In 2014, the group at NMRI reported on a DNA prime/Ad boost malaria vaccine in a phase 1 clinical trial conducted at the WRAIR Clinical Trials Center. The vaccine consisted of three monthly doses of two DNA plasmids encoding CSP and AMA-1 of *P. falciparum* followed four months later by a single boost with a non-replicating Ad5 vector encoding the same genes as the plasmids. Four weeks after the Ad5 boost 15 subjects were challenged with *P. falciparum* sporozoites by mosquito bite, and 4 (27%) were fully protected. No human volunteers with high pre-existing anti-Ad5 neutralizing antibodies were protected.[300] Protection was associated with CD8 T lymphocytes and IFN-γ activities to AMA-1 not CSP. Plasmid DNA priming was required for protection, and subjects immunized with Ad5 alone did not show sterile protection.[301]

Of the many adenoviruses identified in humans, most Ad vaccines use the Ad5 vector, however, because many people around the world have a pre-existing immunity to Ad5 this might limit its usefulness. However, most young children in Africa do not have neutralizing antibodies to Ad5 so this might not preclude its use where falciparum malaria is a principal cause of morbidity and mortality. Because Ad35 is a rare serotype, with a much lower incidence in humans than Ad5, it may provide a more attractive vector. Another alternative to Ad5 and Ad35 is to use the completely foreign (at least to humans) chimpanzee Ad63 (ChAd63).

At the Center for Clinical Vaccinology and Tropical Medicine and Vaccinology, University of Oxford, a phase 1b trial with ChAd63-modified vaccinia Ankara (MVA) virus expressing multiple epitope-thrombospondin related antigenic protein (ME-TRAP) (string consisting mainly of CD8 T lymphocyte epitopes from pre-erythrocytic antigen with TRAP) was used in volunteers in the UK. The ChAd63 ME-TRAP was given intramuscularly and the MVA-ME TRAP was given intradermally 56 days later. Sterile protection against a heterologous strain was found in 3/14 (27%) vaccinees and a delay in the appearance of blood parasites through a reduction of liver stages was observed in 5/14 (36%). Sterile protection and a delay to patency were correlated with production of IFN-γ by CD8 T lymphocytes, not antibody. No sterile efficacy or delay to time in the appearance of blood parasites was observed when there was no MVA boost.[302] In a subsequent study involving a comparison of ChAd63-MVA-CSP with ChAd63-MVA-ME TRAP it was found that only one of 15 vaccinees (17%) receiving the ChAd63 MVA-CSP, and 2/15 (13%) receiving the ChAd63 MVA-ME TRAP achieved sterile protection. Three of the 15 (20%) vaccinees receiving the former and 5/15 (33%) of the latter showed a delay in the time to treatment with antimalarial when compared to controls.[303]

The development of virally vectored vaccinees for malaria is in its early stages and there is still much to be learned from well-designed trials.[304] Future research will have to concentrate on better combinations of antigens and immunization regimens that are safe and reproducibly elicit protective responses in a larger proportion of human volunteers.[301]

A priori the obvious way to develop a protective vaccine for malaria is to employ multiple antigens against several developmental stages of the parasite, however, to date there is no multi-antigen, multi-stage vaccine tested in clinical trials that has been able to induce a strong immune response against each component simultaneously in more than a few volunteers. There is however no shortage of potential vaccine candidates — either composed of a single or several antigens — but of all the vaccine candidates under clinical testing and listed in the 2013 WHO portfolio (Malaria Vaccine Rainbow Tables. http://www.who.int/vaccine_research/ links/Rainbow/en/index.html) most are based on just four antigens (CSP, MSP, TRAP, and AMA) and these were cloned two decades ago. Because there is suggestive evidence that the repeat sequences in CSP and TRAP may act as a smoke screen allowing the malaria parasite to evade the immune response it remains imperative that efforts be directed at identifying other target antigens from among the 5,300 *P. falciparum* putative proteins, however, to date this approach to novel vaccine candidates has been limited.

Chapter 14
Why the Quest Continues

A small number of vaccines exist for an array of bacterial disease such as anthrax, diphtheria, tetanus, typhoid fever, whooping cough (pertussis), pneumococcal pneumonia and meningococcal disease as well as for hepatitis A, hepatitis B, human papilloma virus, influenza, polio, measles, rubella (German measles), shingles, smallpox, chicken pox, yellow fever caused by viruses; however, the number of vaccines against one-celled parasites such as *Plasmodium* (or many-celled parasites such as roundworms and flatworms) is zero. The reasons for this are many.

The successful vaccines for infectious diseases caused by bacteria or their toxic products and viruses are genetically speaking relatively simple pathogens. The number of genes in the influenza virus is eight, mumps has nine, measles 10, for the smallpox virus between 200 and 400 genes, and the protein antigens used for vaccine development i.e. to induce antibodies is relatively small: two for influenza and perhaps several dozen in the case of smallpox.

For smallpox, measles, yellow fever, and the Sabin polio vaccines success was achieved by attenuating the live virus, whereas with the Salk polio vaccine the virulent virus is inactivated by formalin to allow retention of potency and to induce an immune response. In these cases vaccine developers were able to induce antibodies to neutralize key viral proteins. Unfortunately, a similar kind of vaccine will not send the malaria parasite the same way. Indeed, antibody responses are unlikely to afford any protection against the sequestered (intracellular) liver and red blood cell stages of malaria and antibodies may even have a limited effect on the infectious (extracellular) merozoites as they move between cells.

The size and genetic complexity of malaria parasites is many orders of magnitude greater than that of bacteria and viruses. Only since 2002 have researchers been able to look at the complete gene content of malaria parasites to identify potential vaccine candidates from among the 5,300 genes typically found in the lethal *Plasmodium falciparum*. Adding to the complexity is that half of these genes have neither a known function nor a counterpart in any other living creature. Malaria has four different life stages and its own particular mosaic of antigens characterizes each. For example, one study identified 1,289 proteins with 714 present in asexual blood stages, 931 in gametocytes, and 645 in gametes; in another study between 200 and 500 genes were active in salivary gland sporozoites and 246 in gametocytes. Which of these is (are) critical to parasite growth and reproduction is yet to be determined. To build an effective malaria vaccine is tantamount to requiring that the immunization be effective against several microbes simultaneously. Further, malaria parasites, living as they do inside cells, have evolved a series of strategies that allow the *Plasmodium* to confuse, hide, and misdirect the responses of the immune system.

Most of the vaccines under development today were discovered before the genetic blueprint of *P. falciparum* was known and the existing combinations and most in clinical trials are based on just three antigens — circumsporozoite protein (CSP), merozoite surface protein (MSP) and apical membrane antigen (AMA). Unresolved is how antigen combinations should be developed and whether a particular antigen in a combination will interfere with another. There is still no candidate vaccine able to stimulate immunologic memory such that there is long lasting boosting and protection. Often overlooked by those selecting antigens for consideration for incorporation in a vaccine is whether challenging the malaria parasite with a vaccine will result in the emergence of vaccine-resistant mutants.

Another impediment to the development of a malaria vaccine is there appears to be a "species barrier" meaning that although it has been relatively easy to achieve some protection in laboratory mice using a variety of antigens, including DNA-vectored vaccines, adenovirus-vectored vaccines, and prime-boost approaches these have routinely been less than optimal (see p. 226). One explanation for this may be the test system itself: the mouse is not the natural host for the rodent malarias used extensively for testing subunit vaccines or x-irradiated sporozoite vaccines. Some argue that since there is no accepted laboratory correlate of human immunity to malaria and a reliable and predictive animal model does not exist the testing of putative vaccines must be done in human volunteers. The drawbacks of the human challenge model are the time and expenses required to manufacture the vaccine, test its safety, obtain regulatory approval, and then conduct the clinical trial itself. In addition, when vaccine candidates are regarded as failures after a human trial a negative public perception sets in, and this may limit the funding (and enthusiasm) for continued trials. To avoid such a pitfall a great deal of clinical work is often required and much of it has to be done in malaria endemic areas and under strict scientific and ethical standards.

Those vaccine developers who subscribe to the use of monkey models suggest that malaria vaccine trials in non-human primates are less expensive and allow for a choice of antigen before production of clinical grade material. However, monkeys are expensive and there are ecological and ethical concerns about their use. Researchers who reject the use of monkeys argue that it is an invalid model since it uses an unnatural host challenged by an unnatural route and using unnatural dosages. Indeed, in most experimental models of immunity to liver stages very large numbers (50,000–100,000) of x-irradiated sporozoites are injected by intravenous inoculation whereas in nature mosquitoes inoculate a small number (~20 or less) yet we now know sporozoites injected with the mosquito saliva are deposited into the skin and not directly into a blood vessel. These sporozoites move randomly in the skin until they contact the cells lining the capillaries or lymph vessels where they glide around and along until they enter and are carried away rapidly by the blood circulation or more slowly by the lymphatic system. This slow trickling may extend for up to six hour and may lead to a prolonged and very different immune response than parasites injected subcutaneously or directly into the circulation. Indeed, it was shown that much larger numbers of x-irradiated sporozoites were required to elicit the same response through intravenous injection than was induced by the bite of 5–9 irradiated *P. yoelii* infected mosquitoes or by skin injection of 5,000 *x*-irradiated sporozoites. These findings may have a profound bearing on the deployment of a putative malaria vaccine.

Since many of the antigens present in the asexual blood stages are highly variable and may be strain specific a successful protective vaccine must be able to target the invariant regions in the antigen. Such antigens may elicit a reduction in parasite density but can be poorly immunogenic unless coupled with an appropriate adjuvant. There are, however, a limited number of adjuvants available for human use, and Freund's complete adjuvant (FCA) — shown to be very effective in animal models — is not one of them (see p. 69). Formulation of antigens with an adjuvant is empirical as is optimizing the dose and timing of immunizations; all require many time consuming trials and are expensive to carry out. Vaccines designed to block merozoite invasion of red blood cells (see p. 115) by induction of antibodies may be ineffective because the antibodies cannot gain access to the "docking" machinery, or the invasion process itself is completed in a matter of minutes. A further complication is that there may be multiple pathways of invasion available to the parasite so that blocking one simply results in the utilization of an alternate pathway.

There is a current bias in present day vaccines against bacterial and viral diseases in that they contain antigens recognized by antibody. The efficacy of these vaccines is ordinarily measured by their anti-parasitic effect in human subjects in both endemic and non-endemic settings. Nevertheless, there are complications in defining clinical efficacy for a malaria vaccine. What is the critical end-point? Should it be a delay in the appearance of parasites in the blood? Or should it be a reduction in the numbers of parasites in the blood? Should there be sterile immunity? Or, should a reduction in rates of mosquito transmission be the metric? Where will the appropriate clinical trials be held? And, what are the required mosquito transmission rates for assessment of efficacy?

The limited success with protein-based vaccines — ones that usually elicit an antibody response — and the recognition that cell-mediated immunity may be critical for protection against liver and possibly blood stages of malaria has prompted investigations of vaccines that induce strong cell-mediated immunity. Currently, however, none of these vaccines has demonstrated complete protection against a naturally acquired malaria infection and there is little potential for any of them being licensed in the next 5–10 years.

Even when a new malaria vaccine is in hand there may be considerable frustration involved in a scaling up and implementation of vaccination programs as exemplified for the polio and measles vaccines, and for which eradication has not been achieved. Moreover, the economics, financing, marketing, and distributing a pharmaceutical that targets the economically disadvantaged populations of the tropical world where the cost of one series of immunizations might exceed the per capita health spending of the poorest nations represents a formidable challenge.

Realistically, pharmaceutical firms are unlikely to invest the resources necessary to produce a malaria vaccine and satisfy their investors without some promise of a reasonable return on their investment. In the absence of such a commitment, philanthropic and governmental agencies will have to partner with pharmaceutical companies to support the development of malaria vaccines. Such collaborations do exist, as is the case in financing and distributing anti-retroviral therapies to patients in developing countries, however, it remains to be seen whether such cooperation can be maintained for decades while we wait for a fully protective malaria vaccine against humankind's greatest killer. It is for these reasons that it is imperative that the quest continue and that there is assured material support for a new generation of scientists who are prepared to embark on the odyssey.

References

1. White, N. J. *et al.* Malaria. *The Lancet* **383**, 723–735 (2014).
2. Harrison, G. *Mosquitoes, Malaria and Man: A History of Hostilities since 1880*. (Dutton, 1978).
3. Meckel, H. Uber schwartzes Pigment in der Milz und dem blute einer Geisteskranken. *Allg Z Psychiatr Psych Med* **4**, 198–226 (1847).
4. Foster, W. D. in *A History of Parasitology* 158–186 (E and S Livingstone, 1965).
5. Manson-Bahr, P. The story of malaria: the drama and actors. *Int Rev Trop Med* **2**, 329–390 (1963).
6. Kean, B., Mott, K. E. and Russell, A. J. in *Tropical Medicine and Parasitology. Classic Investigations*. **1**, 23–34 (Cornell University Press, 1978).
7. MacCallum, W. G. On the hematozoan infections of birds. *J Exp Med* **3**, 117–135 (1898).
8. De Kruif, P. *Microbe Hunters*. (Harcourt Brace, 1926).
9. Ross, R. *Memoirs: With a Full Account of the Great Malaria Problem and Its Solution*. (Murray, 1923).
10. Bynum, J. and Overy, C. *The Beast in the Mosquito: The Correspondence of Ronald Ross and Patrick Manson*. (Rodopi, 1998).
11. Dobson, M. J. The malariology centenary. *Parassitologia* **41**, 21–32 (1999).
12. Fantini, B. The concept of specificity and the Italian contribution to the discovery of the malaria transmission cycle. *Parassitologia* **41**, 39–47 (1999).
13. Huff, C. G. and Coulston, F. The development of Plasmodium gallinaceum from sporozoite to erythrocytic trophozoite. *J Infect Dis* **75**, 231–249 (1944).
14. Garnham, P. C. C. Exo-erythrocytic schizogony in Plasmodium kochi: a preliminary note. *Trans Roy Soc Trop Med Hyg* **40**, 719–722 (1947).

15. Shortt, H. E. and Garnham, P. C. C. Pre-erythrocytic stage in mammalian malaria parasites. *Nature* **161**, 126 (1948).

16. Coatney, G. R., Collins, W. E., Warren, M. and Contacos, P. G. *The Primate Malarias*. (U.S. Government Printing Office, 1971).

17. Collins, W. E. and Jeffrey, G. M. Plasmodium ovale: parasite and disease. *Clin Microbiol Rev* **18**, 570–581 (2005).

18. Collins, W. E. and Jeffery, G. M. Plasmodium malariae: parasite and disease. *Clin Microbiol Revs* **20**, 579–592 (2007).

19. Shortt, H. E., Fairley, N. H., Covell, G., Shute, P. G. and Garnham, P. C. The pre-erythrocytic stage of Plasmodium falciparum. *Trans R Soc Trop Med Hyg* **44**, 405–419 (1951).

20. Landau, I. and Gautret, P. in *Malaria. Parasite Biology, Pathogenesis and Protection* Sherman, I. W. (ed.) 401–417 (ASM Press, 1998).

21. Krotoski, W. A. The hypnozoite and malarial relapse. *Prog Clin Parasitol* **1**, 1–19 (1989).

22. Greenwood, B. M., Bojang, K., Whitty, C. J. M. and Targett, G. A. T. Malaria. *Lancet* **365**, 1487–1498 (2005).

23. White, N. J. in *Malaria. Parasite Biology, Pathogenesis and Protection* Sherman, I. W. (ed.) 371–385 (ASM Press, 1998).

24. Manwell, R. and Goldstein, F. Passive immunity in avian malaria. *Am J Hyg* **30** (C), 409–421 (1940).

25. Kunkel, Henry G. and Slater, Robert, J. Zone electrophorsis in a starch supporting medium. *Proc Soc Experimental Biol Med* **80**, 42–44 (1952).

26. Makler, M. T., Piper, R. C. and Milhous, W. K. Lactate dehydrogenase and the diagnosis of malaria. *Parasitol Today* **14**, 376–377 (1998).

27. Chiodini, P. L. *et al.* The heat stability of Plasmodium lactate dehydrogenase-based and histidine-rich protein 2-based malaria rapid diagnostic tests. *Trans R Soc Trop Med Hyg* **101**, 331–337 (2007).

28. Tomar, D., Biswas, S., Tripathi, V. and Rao, D. N. Development of diagnostic reagents: raising antibodies against synthetic peptides of PfHRP-2 and LDH using microsphere delivery. *Immunobiology* **211**, 797–805 (2006).

29. Prudhomme, J. and Sherman, I. W. A high capacity *in vitro* assay for measuring the cytoadherence of Plasmodium falciparum infected erythrocytes. *J Immunol Methods* **229**, 169–176 (1999).

30. Seydel, K. B., Milner, D. A., Jr., Kamiza, S. B., Molyneux, M. E. and Taylor, T. E. The distribution and intensity of parasite sequestration in comatose Malawian children. *J Infect Dis* **194**, 208–215 (2006).

31. Stauber, L. A. Some aspects of immunity to intracellular protozoan parasites. *J Parasitol* **49**, 3–11 (1963).

32. Sherman, I. W. Antigens of Plasmodium lophurae. *J Protozool* **11**, 409–417 (1964).
33. Zuckerman, A. Current status of the immunology of malaria and of the antigenic analysis of plasmodia. A five-year review. *Bull World Health Organ* **40**, 55–56 (1969).
34. Zuckerman, A. Current status of the immunology of blood and tissue protozoa. II. Plasmodium. *Exp Parasitol* **42**, 473–446 (1977).
35. Tokuyasu, K., Ilan, J. and Ilan, J. Biogenesis of ribosomes in Plasmodium berghei. *Mil Med* **134**, 1032–1038 (1969).
36. Sherman, I. W., Cox, R. A., Higginson, B., McLaren, D. J. and Williamson, J. The ribosomes of the simian malaria, Plasmodium knowlesi. I. Isolation and characterization. *J Protozool* **22**, 568–572 (1975).
37. Sherman, I. W. The ribosomes of the simian malaria Plasmodium knowlesi — II. A cell-free protein synthesizing system. *Comp Biochem Physiol B* **53**, 447–450 (1976).
38. Sherman, I. W. and Jones, L. A. The Plasmodium lophurae (avian malaria) ribosome. *J Protozool* **24**, 331–334 (1977).
39. Sherman, I. W. Biochemistry of Plasmodium (malarial parasites). *Microbiol Rev* **43**, 453–495 (1979).
40. Jensen, J. B. Reflections on the continuous cultivation of Plasmodium falciparum. *J Parasitol* **91**, 487–491 (2005).
41. Jacobs, H. Immunization against malaria. *Am J Trop Med* **23**, 597–606 (1943).
42. Freund, J. S., H. and Walter, A. Immunization against malaria: vaccination of ducks with killed parasites incorporated with adjuvants. *Science* **102**, 200–202 (1945).
43. Eaton, M. D. and Coggeshall, L. T. Production in monkeys of complement fixing antibodies without active immunity by injection of killed Plasmodium knowlesi. *J Exp Medl* **70**, 141–146 (1939).
44. Heidelberger, M., Coates, W. A. and Mayer, M. Studies in human malaria. II Attempts to influence relapsing vivax malaria by treatment of patients with vaccine (P. vivax). *J Immunol* **52**, 101–107 (1946).
45. Freund, J., Thomson, K. J., Sommer, H. E., Walter, A. W. and Schenkein, E. L. Immunization of rhesus monkeys against malarial infection (p. knowlesi) with killed parasites and adjuvants. *Science* **102**, 202–204 (1945).
46. Freund, J., Thomson, K., Sommer, H., Walter, A. and Pisani, T. Immunization of monkeys against malaria by means of killed parasites with adjuvants. *Am J Trop Med* **28**, 1–22 (1948).

47. Targett, G. A. and Fulton, J. D. Immunization of rhesus monkeys against Plasmodium knowlesi malaria. *Exp Parasitol* **17**, 180–193 (1965).

48. Targett, G. A. and Voller, A. Studies on antibody levels during vaccination of rhesus monkeys against Plasmodium knowlesi. *Br Med J* **2**, 1104–1106 (1965).

49. Kilejian, A. A unique histidine-rich polypeptide from the malarial parasite Plasmodium lophurae. *J Biol Chem* **249**, 4650–4655 (1974).

50. Kilejian, A. Histidine-rich protein as a model malaria vaccine. *Science* **201**, 922–924 (1978).

51. McDonald, V., Hannon, M., Tanigoshi, L. and Sherman, I. W. Plasmodium iophurae: immunization of Pekin ducklings with different antigen preparations. *Exp Parasitol* **51**, 195–203 (1981).

52. Sherman, I. W. Plasmodium lophurae: protective immunogenicity of the histidine-rich protein? *Exp Parasitol* **52**, 292–295 (1981).

53. Kilejian, A. Plasmodium lophurae: immunogenicity of a histidine-rich protein. *Exp Parasitol* **52**, 291 (1981).

54. McGregor, I. A., Gilles, H. M., Walters, J. H., Davies, A. H. and Pearson, F. A. Effects of heavy and repeated malarial infections on Gambian infants and children; effects of erythrocytic parasitization. *Br Med J* **2**, 686–692 (1956).

55. Cohen, S., McGregor, I. and Carrington, S. Gamma-globulin and acquired immunity to human malaria. *Nature* **192**, 733–737 (1961).

56. Butcher, G. A., Cohen, S. and Garnham, P. C. Passive immunity in Plasmodium knowlesi malaria. *Trans R Soc Trop Med Hyg* **64**, 850–856 (1970).

57. Cohen, S., Butcher, G. A. and Crandall, R. B. Action of malarial antibody *in vitro*. *Nature* **223**, 368–371 (1969).

58. Sherman, I. W. *The Elusive Malaria Vaccine. Miracle or Mirage?* (ASM Press, 2009).

59. Anonymous. Editorial. Malaria vaccine on the horizon. *Br Med J* **1**, 231–232 (1975).

60. Siddiqui, W. A. *et al.* Vaccination of experimental monkeys against Plasmodium falciparum: a possible safe adjuvant. *Science* **201**, 1237–1239 (1978).

61. Siddiqui, W. A. in *Malaria*. Kreier, J. (ed.) **3**, 231–262 (Academic, 1980).

62. Desowitz, R. *The Malaria Capers. More Tales of Parasites and People, Research and Reality.* (Norton, 1991).

63. Anonymous. *AID's Malaria Vaccine Research Activities.* 1–55 (General Accounting Office, 1989).

64. Marshall, E. Malaria researcher indicted. *Science* **245**, 1326 (1989).

65. Isikoff, M. *Mismanagement in malaria program.* (Washington Post, 1989).

66. Anonymous. Scientist accused of theft retains post. Science 260, 1415 (1993).
67. Desowitz, R. *Federal Bodysnatchers and the New Guinea Virus.* (Norton, 2002).
68. Yuen, P. C. Recovering funds. *Science* **262**, 164 (1993).
69. Weller, T. *Cultivation of the poliomyelitis virus in tissue culture.* (The Nobel Foundation, 1954).
70. Reese, R. T., Trager, W., Jensen, J. B., Miller, D. A. and Tantravahi, R. Immunization against malaria with antigen from Plasmodium falciparum cultivated *in vitro. Proc Natl Acad Sci USA* **75**, 5665–5668 (1978).
71. Mitchell, G. H., Butcher, G. A. and Cohen, S. Merozoite vaccination against Plasmodium knowlesi malaria. *Immunology* **29**, 397–407 (1975).
72. Mitchell, G. H., Richards, W. H., Voller, A., Dietrich, F. M. and Dukor, P. Nor-MDP, saponin, corynebacteria, and pertussis organisms as immunological adjuvants in experimental malaria vaccination of macaques. *Bull World Health Organ* **57 Suppl 1**, 189–197 (1979).
73. Reese, R. T. and Motyl, M. R. Inhibition of the *in vitro* growth of Plasmodium falciparum. I. The effects of immune serum and purified immunoglobulin from owl monkeys. *J Immunol* **123**, 1894–1899 (1979).
74. Howard, R. F., Varki, A. and Reese, R. T. Merozoite proteins synthesized in P. falciparum schizonts. *Prog Clin Biol Res* **155**, 45–61 (1984).
75. Stanley, H. A. and Reese, R. T. *In vitro* inhibition of intracellular growth of Plasmodium falciparum by immune sera. *Am J Trop Med Hyg* **33**, 12–16 (1984).
76. Stanley, H. A. and Reese, R. T. Monkey-derived monoclonal antibodies against Plasmodium falciparum. *Proc Natl Acad Sci USA* **82**, 6272–6275 (1985).
77. Ardeshir, F., Flint, J. E. and Reese, R. T. Expression of Plasmodium falciparum surface antigens in Escherichia coli. *Proc Natl Acad Sci USA* **82**, 2518–2522 (1985).
78. Ardeshir, F., Flint, J. E., Richman, S. J. and Reese, R. T. A 75 kd merozoite surface protein of Plasmodium falciparum which is related to the 70 kd heat-shock proteins. *Embo J* **6**, 493–499 (1987).
79. Sherman, I. W. *The Malaria Genome Projects: Promise, Progress, and Prospect.* (Imperial College Press, 2012).
80. Sulston, J. and Ferry, G. *The Common Thread. The Story of Science, Politics, Ethics and the Human genome.* (Bantam, 2002).
81. Gardner, M. J. *et al.* Chromosome 2 sequence of the human malaria parasite Plasmodium falciparum. *Science* **282**, 1126–1132 (1998).

82. Bowman, S. *et al.* The complete nucleotide sequence of chromosome 3 of Plasmodium falciparum. *Nature* **400**, 532–538 (1999).
83. Gardner, M. J. *et al.* Genome sequence of the human malaria parasite Plasmodium falciparum. *Nature* **419**, 498–511 (2002).
84. Holt, R. A. *et al.* The genome sequence of the malaria mosquito Anopheles gambiae. *Science* **298**, 129–149 (2002).
85. McGhee, R. Factors affecting the susceptibility of erythrocytes to an intracellular parasite. *Ann N Acad Sci* **56**, 1070–1073 (1953).
86. Sherman, I. W. *In vitro* studies of factors affecting penetration of duck erythrocytes by avian malaria (Plasmodium lophurae). *J Parasitol* **52**, 17–22 (1966).
87. Butcher, G. A., Mitchell, G. H. and Cohen, S. Letter: mechanism of host specificity in malarial infection. *Nature* **244**, 40–41 (1973).
88. Miller, L. H., Mason, S. J., Dvorak, J. A., McGinniss, M. H. and Rothman, I. K. Erythrocyte receptors for (Plasmodium knowlesi) malaria: Duffy blood group determinants. *Science* **189**, 561–563 (1975).
89. Miller, L. H. *et al.* Evidence for differences in erythrocyte surface receptors for the malarial parasites, Plasmodium falciparum and Plasmodium knowlesi. *J Exp Med* **146**, 277–281 (1977).
90. Miller, L. H., Mason, S. J., Clyde, D. F. and McGinniss, M. H. The resistance factor to Plasmodium vivax in blacks. The Duffy-blood-group genotype, FyFy. *N Engl J Med* **295**, 302–304 (1976).
91. Barnwell, J. W., Nichols, M. E. and Rubinstein, P. *In vitro* evaluation of the role of the Duffy blood group in erythrocyte invasion by Plasmodium vivax. *J Exp Med* **169**, 1795–1802 (1989).
92. Tournamille, C., Colin, Y., Cartron, J. P. and Le Van Kim, C. Disruption of a GATA motif in the Duffy gene promoter abolishes erythroid gene expression in Duffy-negative individuals. *Nat Genet* **10**, 224–228 (1995).
93. Cavasini, C. E. *et al.* Plasmodium vivax infection among Duffy antigen-negative individuals from the Brazilian Amazon region: an exception? *Trans R Soc Trop Med Hyg* **101**, 1042–1044 (2007).
94. Ryan, J. R. *et al.* Evidence for transmission of Plasmodium vivax among a Duffy antigen negative population in Western Kenya. *Am J Trop Med Hyg* **75**, 575–581 (2006).
95. Chitnis, C. E. and Miller, L. H. Identification of the erythrocyte binding domains of Plasmodium vivax and Plasmodium knowlesi proteins involved in erythrocyte invasion. *J Exp Med* **180**, 497–506 (1994).
96. Chitnis, C. E. Molecular insights into receptors used by malaria parasites for erythrocyte invasion. *Curr Opin Hematol* **8**, 85–91 (2001).

97. Michon, P., Fraser, T. and Adams, J. H. Naturally acquired and vaccine-elicited antibodies block erythrocyte cytoadherence of the Plasmodium vivax Duffy binding protein. *Infect Immun* **68**, 3164–3171 (2000).

98. King, C. L. *et al.* Naturally acquired Duffy-binding protein-specific binding inhibitory antibodies confer protection from blood-stage Plasmodium vivax infection. *Proc Natl Acad Sci USA* **105**, 8363–8368 (2008).

99. Chitnis, C. E. and Sharma, A. Targeting the Plasmodium vivax Duffy-binding protein. *Trends Parasitol* **24**, 29–34 (2008).

100. Moreno, A. *et al.* Preclinical assessment of the receptor-binding domain of Plasmodium vivax Duffy-binding protein as a vaccine candidate in rhesus macaques. *Vaccine* **26**, 4338–4344 (2008).

101. Ntumngia, F. B., King, C. L. and Adams, J. H. Finding the sweet spots of inhibition: understanding the targets of a functional antibody against Plasmodium vivax Duffy binding protein. *Int J Parasitol* **42**, 1055–1062 (2012).

102. Ntumngia, F. B. *et al.* Immunogenicity of a synthetic vaccine based on Plasmodium vivax Duffy binding protein region II. *Clin Vaccine Immunol CVI* **21**, 1215–1223 (2014).

103. Pasvol, G. and Jungery, M. Glycophorins and red cell invasion by Plasmodium falciparum. *Ciba Found Symp* **94**, 174–195 (1983).

104. Pasvol, G. Receptors on red cells for Plasmodium falciparum and their interaction with merozoites. *Philos Trans R Soc Lond B Biol Sci* **307**, 189–200 (1984).

105. Camus, D. and Hadley, T. J. A Plasmodium falciparum antigen that binds to host erythrocytes and merozoites. *Science* **230**, 553–556 (1985).

106. Duraisingh, M. T., Maier, A. G., Triglia, T. and Cowman, A. F. Erythrocyte-binding antigen 175 mediates invasion in Plasmodium falciparum utilizing sialic acid-dependent and -independent pathways. *Proc Natl Acad Sci USA* **100**, 4796–4801 (2003).

107. Deans, A. M. *et al.* Invasion pathways and malaria severity in Kenyan Plasmodium falciparum clinical isolates. *Infect Immun* **75**, 3014–3020 (2007).

108. Okenu, D. M. *et al.* Analysis of human antibodies to erythrocyte binding antigen 175 of Plasmodium falciparum. *Infect Immun* **68**, 5559–5566 (2000).

109. Richards, J. S. *et al.* Association between naturally acquired antibodies to erythrocyte-binding antigens of Plasmodium falciparum and protection from malaria and high-density parasitemia. *Clin Infect Dis* **51**, e50–e60 (2010).

110. Badiane, A. S. *et al.* Inhibitory humoral responses to the Plasmodium falciparum vaccine candidate EBA-175 are independent of the erythrocyte invasion pathway. *Clin Vaccine Immunol CVI* **20**, 1238–1245 (2013).

111. Healer, J. *et al.* Vaccination with conserved regions of erythrocyte-binding antigens induces neutralizing antibodies against multiple strains of Plasmodium falciparum. *PloS One* **8**, e72504 (2013).

112. El Sahly, H. M. *et al.* Safety and immunogenicity of a recombinant nonglycosylated erythrocyte binding antigen 175 Region II malaria vaccine in healthy adults living in an area where malaria is not endemic. *Clin Vaccine Immunol CVI* **17**, 1552–1559 (2010).

113. Wanaguru, M., Crosnier, C., Johnson, S., Rayner, J. C. and Wright, G. J. Biochemical analysis of the Plasmodium falciparum erythrocyte-binding antigen-175 (EBA175)-glycophorin-A interaction: implications for vaccine design. *J Biol Chem* **288**, 32106–32117 (2013).

114. Freeman, R. R., Trejdosiewicz, A. J. and Cross, G. A. Protective monoclonal antibodies recognising stage-specific merozoite antigens of a rodent malaria parasite. *Nature* **284**, 366–368 (1980).

115. Holder, A. A. and Freeman, R. R. Immunization against blood-stage rodent malaria using purified parasite antigens. *Nature* **294**, 361–364 (1981).

116. Holder, A. A., Freeman, R. R. and Nicholls, S. C. Immunization against Plasmodium falciparum with recombinant polypeptides produced in Escherichia coli. *Parasite Immunol* **10**, 607–617 (1988).

117. Holder, A. A. *et al.* Merozoite surface protein 1, immune evasion, and vaccines against asexual blood stage malaria. *Parassitologia* **41**, 409–414 (1999).

118. Blackman, M. J., Scott-Finnigan, T. J., Shai, S. and Holder, A. A. Antibodies inhibit the protease-mediated processing of a malaria merozoite surface protein. *J Exp Med* **180**, 389–393 (1994).

119. Singh, S. *et al.* Immunity to recombinant plasmodium falciparum merozoite surface protein 1 (MSP1): protection in Aotus nancymai monkeys strongly correlates with anti-MSP1 antibody titer and *in vitro* parasite-inhibitory activity. *Infect Immun* **74**, 4573–4580 (2006).

120. Stowers, A. W. *et al.* Efficacy of two alternate vaccines based on Plasmodium falciparum merozoite surface protein 1 in an Aotus challenge trial. *Infect Immun* **69**, 1536–1546 (2001).

121. Stoute, J. A. *et al.* Phase 1 randomized double-blind safety and immunogenicity trial of Plasmodium falciparum malaria merozoite surface protein FMP1 vaccine, adjuvanted with AS02A, in adults in western Kenya. *Vaccine* **25**, 176–184 (2007).

122. Otsyula, N. *et al.* Results from tandem Phase 1 studies evaluating the safety, reactogenicity and immunogenicity of the vaccine candidate antigen Plasmodium falciparum FVO merozoite surface protein-1 (MSP1(42)) administered intramuscularly with adjuvant system AS01. *Malar J* **12**, 29 (2013).

123. Deans, J. Protective antigens of blood stage Plasmodium knowelsi parasites. *Phil Trans R Soc Lond B* **307**, 159–169 (1984).

124. Deans, J. A. *et al.* Rat monoclonal antibodies which inhibit the *in vitro* multiplication of Plasmodium knowlesi. *Clin Exp Immunol* **49**, 297–309 (1982).

125. Mitchell, G. H., Thomas, A. W., Margos, G., Dluzewski, A. R. and Bannister, L. H. Apical membrane antigen 1, a major malaria vaccine candidate, mediates the close attachment of invasive merozoites to host red blood cells. *Infect Immun* **72**, 154–158 (2004).

126. Deans, J. A. *et al.* Vaccination trials in rhesus monkeys with a minor, invariant, Plasmodium knowlesi 66 kD merozoite antigen. *Parasite Immunol* **10**, 535–552 (1988).

127. Peterson, M. G. *et al.* Integral membrane protein located in the apical complex of Plasmodium falciparum. *Mol Cell Biol* **9**, 3151–3154 (1989).

128. Kemp, D. J. *et al.* Expression of Plasmodium falciparum blood-stage antigens in Escherichia coli: detection with antibodies from immune humans. *Proc Natl Acad Sci USA* **80**, 3787–3791 (1983).

129. Brown, G. V. *et al.* The expression of Plasmodium falciparum bloodstage antigens in Escherichia coli. *Philos Trans R Soc Lond B Biol Sci* **307**, 179–187 (1984).

130. Cowman, A. F. *et al.* Conserved sequences flank variable tandem repeats in two S-antigen genes of Plasmodium falciparum. *Cell* **40**, 775–783 (1985).

131. Cowman, A. F. *et al.* The ring-infected erythrocyte surface antigen (RESA) polypeptide of Plasmodium falciparum contains two separate blocks of tandem repeats encoding antigenic epitopes that are naturally immunogenic in man. *Mol Biol Med* **2**, 207–221 (1984).

132. Harvey, K. L., Gilson, P. R. and Crabb, B. S. A model for the progression of receptor-ligand interactions during erythrocyte invasion by Plasmodium falciparum. *Int J Parasitol* **42**, 567–573 (2012).

133. Remarque, E., Faber, B., Kocken, C. and Thomas, A. Apical memebrane antigen 1: a malaria vaccine candidate. *Trends Parasitol* **24**, 74–84 (2007).

134. Saul, A. *et al.* A human phase 1 vaccine clinical trial of the Plasmodium falciparum malaria vaccine candidate apical membrane antigen 1 in Montanide ISA720 adjuvant. *Vaccine* **23**, 3076–3083 (2005).

135. Malkin, E. M. *et al.* Phase 1 clinical trial of apical membrane antigen 1: an asexual blood-stage vaccine for Plasmodium falciparum malaria. *Infect Immun* **73**, 3677–3685 (2005).

136. Thera, M. A. *et al.* Safety and immunogenicity of an AMA-1 malaria vaccine in Malian adults: results of a phase 1 randomized controlled trial. *PLoS ONE* **3**, e1465 (2008).

137. Schussek, S. *et al.* Immunization with apical membrane antigen 1 confers sterile infection-blocking immunity against Plasmodium sporozoite challenge in a rodent model. *Infect Immun* **81**, 3586–3599 (2013).

138. Cowman, A. F. and Crabb, B. S. Invasion of red blood cells by malaria parasites. *Cell* **124**, 755–766 (2006).

139. Crosnier, C. *et al.* Basigin is a receptor essential for erythrocyte invasion by Plasmodium falciparum. *Nature* **480**, 534–537 (2011).

140. Bustamante, L. Y. *et al.* A full-length recombinant Plasmodium falciparum PfRH5 protein induces inhibitory antibodies that are effective across common PfRH5 genetic variants. *Vaccine* **31**, 373–379 (2013).

141. Reddy, K. S. *et al.* Multiprotein complex between the GPI-anchored CyRPA with PfRH5 and PfRipr is crucial for Plasmodium falciparum erythrocyte invasion. *Proc Natl Acad Sci USA* **112**, 1179–1184 (2015).

142. Tran, T. M. *et al.* Naturally acquired antibodies specific for Plasmodium falciparum reticulocyte-binding protein homologue 5 inhibit parasite growth and predict protection from malaria. *J Infect Dis* **209**, 789–798 (2014).

143. Douglas, A. D. *et al.* A PfRH5-based vaccine is efficacious against Heterologous strain blood-stage Plasmodium falciparum infection in aotus monkeys. *Cell Host Microbe* **17**, 130–139 (2015).

144. Dreyer, A. M. *et al.* Passive immunoprotection of Plasmodium falciparum-infected mice designates the CyRPA as candidate malaria vaccine antigen. *J Immunol Baltim Md 1950* **188**, 6225–6237 (2012).

145. Chen, L. *et al.* An EGF-like protein forms a complex with PfRh5 and is required for invasion of human erythrocytes by Plasmodium falciparum. *PLoS Pathog* **7**, e1002199 (2011).

146. Tham, W.-H., Healer, J. and Cowman, A. F. Erythrocyte and reticulocyte binding-like proteins of Plasmodium falciparum. *Trends Parasitol* **28**, 23–30 (2012).

147. Patarroyo, M. E. *et al.* Induction of protective immunity against experimental infection with malaria using synthetic peptides. *Nature* **328**, 629–32 (1987).

148. Brooke, J. *Colombian physician challenges malaria on the home front.* (NY Times, 1993).

149. Patarroyo, M. E. *et al.* A synthetic vaccine protects humans against challenge with asexual blood stages of Plasmodium falciparum malaria. *Nature* **332**, 158–61 (1988).

150. Maurice, J. Controversial vaccine shows promise. *Science* **259**, 1689–1690 (1993).

151. Valero, M. V. *et al.* Vaccination with SPf66, a chemically synthesised vaccine, against Plasmodium falciparum malaria in Colombia. *Lancet* **341**, 705–710 (1993).

152. Marshall, E. Serious setback for Patarroyo. *Science* **273**, 1652 (1996).

153. Trager, W. Malaria vaccine. *Science* **267**, 1577 (1995).

154. Alonso, P. L. *et al.* Randomised trial of efficacy of SPf66 vaccine against Plasmodium falciparum malaria in children in southern Tanzania. *Lancet* **344**, 1175–1181 (1994).

155. Graves, P., Gelband, H. and Garner, P. The SPf66 malaria vaccine: what is the evidence for efficacy? *Parasitol Today* **14**, 218–220 (1998).

156. Bojang, K. A. *et al.* An efficacy trial of the malaria vaccine SPf66 in Gambian infants — second year of follow-up. *Vaccine* **16**, 62–67 (1998).

157. Acosta, C. J. *et al.* Evaluation of the SPf66 vaccine for malaria control when delivered through the EPI scheme in Tanzania. *Trop Med Int Health* **4**, 368–376 (1999).

158. Druilhe, P. and Marchand, C. in *Frontiers of infectious diseases. New strategies in parasitology McAdams*, K. P. W. (ed.) 39–50 (Churchill Livingstone, 1989).

159. Druilhe, P., Renia, L. and Fidock, D. in *Malaria. Parsite biology, pathogenesis and protection* Sherman, I. W. (ed.) 513–544 (ASM Press, 1998).

160. Khusmith, S., Druilhe, P. and Gentilini, M. [Activity of monocytes of subjects sensitized to Plasmodium falciparum: adherence and phagocytosis of merozoites *in vitro*. Role of cytophylic antibodies]. *Bull Société Pathol Exot Ses Fil* **76**, 137–145 (1983).

161. Druilhe, P. and Barnwell, J. W. Pre-erythrocytic stage malaria vaccines: time for a change in path. *Curr Opin Microbiol* **10**, 371–378 (2007).

162. Bouharoun-Tayoun, H., Attanath, P., Sabchareon, A., Chongsuphajaisiddhi, T. and Druilhe, P. Antibodies that protect humans against Plasmodium falciparum blood stages do not on their own inhibit parasite growth and invasion *in vitro*, but act in cooperation with monocytes. *J. Exp. Med.* **172**, 1633–1641 (1990).

163. Oeuvray, C. *et al.* Merozoite surface protein-3: a malaria protein inducing antibodies that promote Plasmodium falciparum killing by cooperation with blood monocytes. *Blood* **84**, 1594–1602 (1994).

164. Bang, G., Prieur, E., Roussilhon, C. and Druilhe, P. Pre-clinical assessment of novel multivalent MSP3 malaria vaccine constructs. *PloS One* **6**, e28165 (2011).

165. Sirima, S. B., Cousens, S. and Druilhe, P. Protection against malaria by MSP3 candidate vaccine. *N Engl J Med* **365**, 1062–1064 (2011).

166. Bitencourt, A. R. *et al.* Antigenicity and immunogenicity of Plasmodium vivax merozoite surface protein-3. *PloS One* **8**, e56061 (2013).

167. Theisen, M. *et al.* A Plasmodium falciparum GLURP-MSP3 chimeric protein; expression in Lactococcus lactis, immunogenicity and induction of biologically active antibodies. *Vaccine* **22**, 1188–1198 (2004).

168. Jepsen, M. P. G. *et al.* The malaria vaccine candidate GMZ2 elicits functional antibodies in individuals from malaria endemic and non-endemic areas. *J Infect Dis* **208**, 479–488 (2013).

169. Takahashi, Y. and Sherman, I. W. Plasmodium iophurae: cationized ferritin staining, an electron microscope cytochemical method for differentiating malarial parasite and host cell membranes. *Exp Parasitol* **44**, 145–154 (1978).

170. Bignami, A. and Bastianelli, G. Observazioni suile febbri malariche estive-autunnali. *Riforma Med* **232**, 1334–1335 (1890).

171. Gruenberg, J. and Sherman, I. W. Isolation and characterization of the plasma membrane of human erythrocytes infected with the malarial parasite Plasmodium falciparum. *Proc Natl Acad Sci USA* **80**, 1087–1091 (1983).

172. Trager, W., Rudzinska, M. A. and Bradbury, P. C. The fine structure of Plasmodium falciparum and its host erythrocytes in natural malarial infections in man. *Bull World Health Organ* **35**, 883–885 (1966).

173. Luse, S. A. and Miller, L. H. Plasmodium falciparum malaria. Ultrastructure of parasitized erythrocytes in cardiac vessels. *Am J Trop Med Hyg* **20**, 655–660 (1971).

174. Miller, L. H. The ultrastructure of red cells infected by Plasmodium falciparum in man. *Trans R Soc Trop Med Hyg* **66**, 459–462 (1972).

175. Langreth, S. G., Jensen, J. B., Reese, R. T. and Trager, W. Fine structure of human malaria *in vitro*. *J Protozool* **25**, 443–452 (1978).

176. Udeinya, I. J., Schmidt, J. A., Aikawa, M., Miller, L. H. and Green, I. Falciparum malaria-infected erythrocytes specifically bind to cultured human endothelial cells. *Science* **213**, 555–557 (1981).

177. Langreth, S. G. and Reese, R. T. Antigenicity of the infected-erythrocyte and merozoite surfaces in Falciparum malaria. *J Exp Med* **150**, 1241–1254 (1979).

178. Eaton, M. D. the agglutination of Plasmodium knowlesi by immune serum. *J Exp Med* **67**, 857 (1938).

179. Brown, K. N. and Brown, I. N. Immunity to malaria: antigenic variation in chronic infections of Plasmodium knowlesi. *Nature* **208**, 1286–1288 (1965).

180. Brown, K. N. Antibody-induced variation in malaria parasites. *Nature* **242**, 49–50 (1973).

181. Brown, K. N. in *Immunology of Parasitic Infections* Cohen, S. and Sadun, E. (eds.) (Blackwell, 1976).

182. Brown, K. N., Brown, I. N. and Hills, L. A. Immunity to malaria. I. Protection against Plasmodium knowlesi shown by monkeys sensitized with drug-suppressed infections or by dead parasites in Freund's adjuvant. *Exp Parasitol* **28**, 304–317 (1970).

183. Butcher, G. A. and Cohen, S. Antigenic variation and protective immunity in Plasmodium knowlesi malaria. *Immunology* **23**, 503–21 (1972).

184. Barnwell, J. W., Howard, R. J., Coon, H. G. and Miller, L. H. Splenic requirement for antigenic variation and expression of the variant antigen on the erythrocyte membrane in cloned Plasmodium knowlesi malaria. *Infect Immun* **40**, 985–994 (1983).

185. Boyle, D. B., March, J. C., Newbold, C. I. and Brown, K. N. Parasite polypeptides lost during schizogony and erythrocyte invasion by the malaria parasites, Plasmodium chabaudi and Plasmodium knowlesi. *Mol Biochem Parasitol* **7**, 9–18 (1983).

186. Howard, R. J., Barnwell, J. W., Kao, V., Daniel, W. A. and Aley, S. B. Radioiodination of new protein antigens on the surface of Plasmodium knowlesi schizont-infected erythrocytes. *Mol Biochem Parasitol* **6**, 343–367 (1982).

187. Leech, J. H., Barnwell, J. W., Miller, L. H. and Howard, R. J. Identification of a strain-specific malarial antigen exposed on the surface of Plasmodium falciparum-infected erythrocytes. *J Exp Med* **159**, 1567–1575 (1984).

188. Baruch, D. I. *et al.* Cloning the P. falciparum gene encoding PfEMP1, a malarial variant antigen and adherence receptor on the surface of parasitized human erythrocytes. *Cell* **82**, 77–87 (1995).

189. Smith, J. D. *et al.* Switches in expression of Plasmodium falciparum var genes correlate with changes in antigenic and cytoadherent phenotypes of infected erythrocytes. *Cell* **82**, 101–110 (1995).

190. Su, X. Z. *et al.* The large diverse gene family var encodes proteins involved in cytoadherence and antigenic variation of Plasmodium falciparum-infected erythrocytes. *Cell* **82**, 89–100 (1995).

191. Guizetti, J. and Scherf, A. Silence, activate, poise and switch! Mechanisms of antigenic variation in Plasmodium falciparum. *Cell Microbiol* **15**, 718–726 (2013).

192. Smith, J. D. The role of PfEMP1 adhesion domain classification in Plasmodium falciparum pathogenesis research. *Mol Biochem Parasitol* **195**, 82–87 (2014).

193. Scherf, A., Lopez-Rubio, J. J. and Riviere, L. Antigenic Variation in Plasmodium falciparum. *Annu Rev Microbiol* **62**, 445–470 (2008).

194. Baruch, D. I. Adhesive receptors on malaria-parasitized red cells. *Baillieres Best Pr Res Clin Haematol* **12**, 747–761 (1999).

195. Baruch, D. I., Gamain, B. and Miller, L. H. DNA immunization with the cysteine-rich interdomain region 1 of the Plasmodium falciparum variant antigen elicits limited cross-reactive antibody responses. *Infect Immun* **71**, 4536–4543 (2003).

196. Gratepanche, S. *et al.* Induction of crossreactive antibodies against the Plasmodium falciparum variant protein. *Proc Natl Acad Sci USA* **100**, 13007–13012 (2003).

197. Locher, C. P., Paidhungat, M., Whalen, R. G. and Punnonen, J. DNA shuffling and screening strategies for improving vaccine efficacy. *DNA Cell Biol* **24**, 256–263 (2005).

198. Storm, J. and Craig, A. G. Pathogenesis of cerebral malaria — inflammation and cytoadherence. *Front Cell Infect Microbiol* **4**, 100 (2014).

199. Lau, C. K. Y. *et al.* Structural conservation despite huge sequence diversity allows EPCR binding by the PfEMP1 family implicated in severe childhood malaria. *Cell Host Microbe* **17**, 118–129 (2015).

200. Fairhurst, R. M. PfEMP1's magical embrace of EPCR. *Cell Host Microbe* **17**, 10–12 (2015).

201. Cabrera, A., Neculai, D. and Kain, K. C. CD36 and malaria: friends or foes? A decade of data provides some answers. *Trends Parasitol* **30**, 436–444 (2014).

202. Fry, A. E. *et al.* Positive selection of a CD36 nonsense variant in sub-Saharan Africa, but no association with severe malaria phenotypes. *Hum Mol Genet* **18**, 2683–2692 (2009).

203. Fried, M. *et al.* Multilaboratory approach to preclinical evaluation of vaccine immunogens for placental malaria. *Infect Immun* **81**, 487–495 (2013).

204. Saveria, T. *et al.* Antibodies to Escherichia coli-expressed C-terminal domains of Plasmodium falciparum variant surface antigen 2-chondroitin sulfate A (VAR2CSA) inhibit binding of CSA-adherent parasites to placental tissue. *Infect Immun* **81**, 1031–1039 (2013).

205. Bigey, P. *et al.* The NTS-DBL2X region of VAR2CSA induces cross-reactive antibodies that inhibit adhesion of several Plasmodium falciparum isolates to chondroitin sulfate A. *J Infect Dis* **204**, 1125–1133 (2011).

206. Gruenberg, J., Allred, D. R. and Sherman, I. W. Scanning electron microscope-analysis of the protrusions (knobs) present on the surface of Plasmodium falciparum-infected erythrocytes. *J Cell Biol* **97**, 795–802 (1983).

207. Howard, R. J. *Malaria and the Red Cell* (Ciba Foundation Symposium 94), D. Evered and J. Whelan (eds.) p. 237 (Pitman, London, 1983).

208. Winograd, E. and Sherman, I. W. Characterization of a modified red cell membrane protein expressed on erythrocytes infected with the human malaria parasite Plasmodium falciparum: possible role as a cytoadherent mediating protein. *J Cell Biol* **108**, 23–30 (1989).

209. Crandall, I. and Sherman, I. W. Antibodies to synthetic peptides based on band 3 motifs react specifically with Plasmodium falciparum (human malaria)-infected erythrocytes and block cytoadherence. *Parasitology* **108 (Pt 4)**, 389–396 (1994).

210. Crandall, I., Collins, W. E., Gysin, J. and Sherman, I. W. Synthetic peptides based on motifs present in human band 3 protein inhibit cytoadherence/sequestration of the malaria parasite Plasmodium falciparum. *Proc Natl Acad Sci USA* **90**, 4703–4707 (1993).

211. Hogh, B., Petersen, E., Crandall, I., Gottschau, A. and Sherman, I. W. Immune responses to band 3 neoantigens on Plasmodium falciparum-infected erythrocytes in subjects living in an area of intense malaria transmission are associated with low parasite density and high hematocrit value. *Infect Immun* **62**, 4362–4366 (1994).

212. Guthrie, N., Bird, D. M., Crandall, I. and Sherman, I. W. Plasmodium falciparum: the adherence of erythrocytes infected with human malaria can be mimicked using pfalhesin-coated microspheres. *Cell Adhes Commun* **3**, 407–417 (1995).

213. Winograd, E., Eda, S. and Sherman, I. W. Chemical modifications of band 3 protein affect the adhesion of Plasmodium falciparum-infected erythrocytes to CD36. *Mol Biochem Parasitol* **136**, 243–248 (2004).

214. Winograd, E. and Sherman, I. W. Malaria infection induces a conformational change in erythrocyte band 3 protein. *Mol Biochem Parasitol* **138**, 83–87 (2004).

215. Kennedy, J. R. Malaria: a vaccine concept based on sickle haemoglobin's augmentation of an innate autoimmune process to band 3. *Int J Parasitol* **31**, 1275–1277 (2001).

216. Eyles, D. Studies on Plasmodium gallinaceum. I. Factors associated with the malaria infection in the vertebrate host which influence the degree of infection in the mosquito. *Am J Hyg* **55**, 386–391 (1952).

217. Eyles, D. Studies on Plasmodium gallinaceum. II. Factors in the blood of the vertebrate host influencing mosquito infection. *Am J Hyg* **55**, 276–290 (1952).

218. Gwadz, R. W. Successful immunization against the sexual stages of Plasmodium gallinaceum. *Science* **193**, 1150–1151 (1976).

219. Carter, R. and Chen, D. H. Malaria transmission blocked by immunisation with gametes of the malaria parasite. *Nature* **263**, 57–60 (1976).

220. Vermeulen, A. N. *et al.* Characterization of Plasmodium falciparum sexual stage antigens and their biosynthesis in synchronised gametocyte cultures. *Mol Biochem Parasitol* **20**, 155–163 (1986).

221. Williamson, K. C. Pfs 230: from malaria transmission-blocking vaccine candidate toward function. *Parasite Immunol* **25**, 351–359 (2003).

222. Pradel, G. Proteins of the malaria parasite sexual stages: expression, function and potential for transmission blocking strategies. *Parasitology* **134**, 1911–1929 (2007).

223. Vermeulen, A. N. *et al.* Sequential expression of antigens on sexual stages of Plasmodium falciparum accessible to transmission-blocking antibodies in the mosquito. *J Exp Med* **162**, 1460–1476 (1985).

224. Outchkourov, N. S. *et al.* Correctly folded Pfs48/45 protein of Plasmodium falciparum elicits malaria transmission-blocking immunity in mice. *Proc Natl Acad Sci USA* **105**, 4301–4305 (2008).

225. Carter, R., Gwadz, R. W. and McAuliffe, F. M. Plasmodium gallinaceum: transmission-blocking immunity in chickens. I. Comparative immunogenicity of gametocyte- and gamete-containing preparations. *Exp Parasitol* **47**, 185–193 (1979).

226. Gwadz, R. W. and Koontz, L. C. Plasmodium knowlesi: persistence of transmission blocking immunity in monkeys immunized with gamete antigens. *Infect Immun* **44**, 137–140 (1984).

227. Gamage-Mendis, A. C., Rajakaruna, J., Carter, R. and Mendis, K. N. Transmission blocking immunity to human Plasmodium vivax malaria in an endemic population in Kataragama, Sri Lanka. *Parasite Immunol* **14**, 385–396 (1992).

228. Graves, P. M., Carter, R., Burkot, T. R., Quakyi, I. A. and Kumar, N. Antibodies to Plasmodium falciparum gamete surface antigens in Papua New Guinea sera. *Parasite Immunol* **10**, 209–218 (1988).

229. Grotendorst, C. A., Kumar, N., Carter, R. and Kaushal, D. C. A surface protein expressed during the transformation of zygotes of Plasmodium gallinaceum is a target of transmission-blocking antibodies. *Infect Immun* **45**, 775–777 (1984).

230. Carter, R. and Kaushal, D. C. Characterization of antigens on mosquito midgut stages of Plasmodium gallinaceum. III. Changes in zygote surface proteins during transformation to mature ookinete. *Mol Biochem Parasitol* **13**, 235–241 (1984).

231. Kumar, N. and Carter, R. Biosynthesis of two stage-specific membrane proteins during transformation of Plasmodium gallinaceum zygotes into ookinetes. *Mol Biochem Parasitol* **14**, 127–139 (1985).

232. Kaslow, D. C. in *Malaria Vaccine Development* Hoffman, S. L. (ed.) (ASM Press, 1996).

233. Kaslow, D. C. in *Vaccines: from Concept to Clinic* Paoletti, L. C. and McInnes, P. M. (eds.) (CRC Press, 1999).

234. Kaslow, D. C. Malaria immunology. in *Chemical Immunol* Perlmann, P. and Troye-Blomberg, M. (eds.) **80**, 287–307 (Basel, Karger, 2002).

235. Wu, Y. *et al.* Phase 1 trial of malaria transmission blocking vaccine candidates Pfs25 and Pvs25 formulated with montanide ISA 51. *PLoS ONE* **3**, e2636 (2008).

236. Lobo, C. A., Dhar, R. and Kumar, N. Immunization of mice with DNA-based Pfs25 elicits potent malaria transmission-blocking antibodies. *Infect Immun* **67**, 1688–1693 (1999).

237. Shimp, R. L. *et al.* Development of a Pfs25-EPA malaria transmission blocking vaccine as a chemically conjugated nanoparticle. *Vaccine* **31**, 2954–2962 (2013).

238. Jones, R. M. *et al.* A plant-produced Pfs25 VLP malaria vaccine candidate induces persistent transmission blocking antibodies against Plasmodium falciparum in immunized mice. *PloS One* **8**, e79538 (2013).

239. Mulligan, H. W., Russell, P. F. and Mohan, B. N. Active immunization of fowls against Plasmodium gallinaceum by injections of killed homologous sporozoites. *J Mal Inst India* **4**, 25–34 (1941).

240. Radke, M. and Sadun, E. H. Resistance produced in mice by exposure to irradiated Schistosoma mansoni cercariae. *Exp Parasitol* **13**, 134–142 (1963).

241. Hsu, S., Hsu, H. F. and Burmeister, L. F. Schistosoma mansoni: vaccination of mice with highly x-irradiated cercariae. *Exp Parasitol* **52**, 91–104 (1981).

242. Nussenzweig, R. S., Vanderberg, J., Most, H. and Orton, C. Protective immunity produced by the injection of x-irradiated sporozoites of Plasmodium berghei. *Nature* **216**, 160–162 (1967).

243. Verhave, J. P. *Immunization with sporozoites: An experimental study of Plasmodium berghei malaria*. (Catholic University, 1975).
244. Orjih, A. U., Cochrane, A. H. and Nussenzweig, R. S. Comparative studies on the immunogenicity of infective and attenuated sporozoites of Plasmodium berghei. *Trans R Soc Trop Med Hyg* **76**, 57–61 (1982).
245. Vanderberg, J., Nussenzweig, R. and Most, H. Protective immunity produced by the injection of x-irradiated sporozoites of Plasmodium berghei. V. *In vitro* effects of immune serum on sporozoites. *Mil Med* **134**, 1183–1190 (1969).
246. Cochrane, A. H., Nussenzweig, R. and Nardin, E. in *Malaria* (ed. Kreier, J.) **3**, 163–202 (Academic Press, 1980).
247. Oransky, I. David Francis Clyde. *Lancet* **361**, 439 (2003).
248. Clyde, D. F. Immunity to falciparum and vivax malaria induced by irradiated sporozoites: a review of the University of maryland studies 1971–1975. *Bull World Health Organ* **68 (Suppl 1)**, 9–12 (1990).
249. Rieckmann, K. H. Human immunization with attenuated sporozoites. *Bull World Health Organ* **68 (Suppl 1)**, 13–16 (1990).
250. Vanderberg, J., Nussenzweig, R. and Most, H. Protective immunity produced by the bite of x-irradiated mosquitoes infected with Plasmodium berghei. *J Parasitol* **56**, 350–351 (1970).
251. Clyde, D. F. Immunization of man against falciparum and vivax malaria by use of attenuated sporozoites. *Am J Trop Med Hyg* **24**, 397–401 (1975).
252. Altman, L. K. *Who Goes First? The Story of Self-Experimentation in Medicine*. (Random House, 1987).
253. Yoshida, N., Nussenzweig, R. S., Potocnjak, P., Nussenzweig, V. and Aikawa, M. Hybridoma produces protective antibodies directed against the sporozoite stage of malaria parasite. *Science* **207**, 71–73 (1980).
254. Ellis, J. *et al.* Cloning and expression in E. coli of the malarial sporozoite surface antigen gene from Plasmodium knowlesi. *Nature* **302**, 536–538 (1983).
255. Dame, J. B. *et al.* Structure of the gene encoding the immunodominant surface antigen on the sporozoite of the human malaria parasite Plasmodium falciparum. *Science* **225**, 593–599 (1984).
256. Enea, V. *et al.* Circumsporozoite gene of Plasmodium cynomolgi (Gombak): cDNA cloning and expression of the repetitive circumsporozoite epitope. *Proc Natl Acad Sci USA* **81**, 7520–7524 (1984).
257. Lal, A. A. *et al.* Structure of the circumsporozoite gene of Plasmodium malariae. *Mol Biochem Parasitol* **30**, 291–294 (1988).

258. McCutchan, T. F. *et al.* Sequence of the immunodominant epitope for the surface protein on sporozoites of Plasmodium vivax. *Science* **230**, 1381–1383 (1985).

259. Boffey, P. M. Malaria vaccine is near, U.S. health officials say. *NY Times* (1984).

260. Herrington, D. A. *et al.* Safety and immunogenicity of a recombinant sporozoite malaria vaccine against Plasmodium vivax. *Am J Trop Med Hyg* **45**, 695–701 (1991).

261. Hoffman, S. L., Sedegah, M. and Hedstrom, R. C. Protection against malaria by immunization with a Plasmodium yoelii circumsporozoite protein nucleic acid vaccine. *Vaccine* **12**, 1529–1533 (1994).

262. Ballou, W. R. *et al.* Safety and efficacy of a recombinant DNA Plasmodium falciparum sporozoite vaccine. *Lancet* **1**, 1277–1281 (1987).

263. Sinnis, P. and Nussenzweig, V. in *Malaria Vaccine Development: a Multi-Immune Response Approach* Hoffman, S. (ed.) 15–33 (ASM Press, 1996).

264. Sadun, E. H. Introduction to the International Panel Workshop on Biological Research in Malaria. *Mil Med* **131**, Suppl: 847–852 (1966).

265. Weinstein, P. P. In memoriam. Elvio Herbert Sadun. *J Parasitol* **40**, 897–899 (1974).

266. Wellde, B. T., Diggs, C. L. and Anderson, S. Immunization of Aotus trivirgatus against Plasmodium falciparum with irradiated blood forms. *Bull World Health Organ* **57 Suppl 1**, 153–157 (1979).

267. Diggs, C. L., Hines, F. and Wellde, B. T. Plasmodium falciparum: passive immunization of Aotus lemurinus griseimembra with immune serum. *Exp Parasitol* **80**, 291–296 (1995).

268. Haynes, J. D., Diggs, C. L., Hines, F. A. and Desjardins, R. E. Culture of human malaria parasites Plasmodium falciparum. *Nature* **263**, 767–769 (1976).

269. Ballou, W. R. Obstacles to the development of a safe and effective attenuated pre-erythrocytic stage malaria vaccine. *Microbes Infect* **9**, 761–766 (2007).

270. Heppner, D. G. *et al.* Safety, immunogenicity, and efficacy of Plasmodium falciparum repeatless circumsporozoite protein vaccine encapsulated in liposomes. *J Infect Dis* **174**, 361–366 (1996).

271. Cohen, J., Nussenzweig, V., Nussenzweig, R., Vekemans, J. and Leach, A. From the circumsporozoite protein to the RTS, S/AS candidate vaccine. *Hum Vaccin* **6**, 90–96 (2010).

272. Gordon, D. M. *et al.* Safety, immunogenicity, and efficacy of a recombinantly produced Plasmodium falciparum circumsporozoite protein-hepatitis B surface antigen subunit vaccine. *J Infect Dis* **171**, 1576–1585 (1995).

273. Heppner, D. G., Jr. *et al.* Towards an RTS, S-based, multi-stage, multi-antigen vaccine against falciparum malaria: progress at the Walter Reed Army Institute of Research. *Vaccine* **23**, 2243–2250 (2005).

274. Stoute, J. A. *et al.* A preliminary evaluation of a recombinant circumsporozoite protein vaccine against Plasmodium falciparum malaria. RTS, S malaria vaccine evaluation group. *N Engl J Med* **336**, 86–91 (1997).

275. Ballou, W. R. and Cahill, C. P. Two decades of commitment to malaria vaccine development: GlaxoSmithKline biologicals. *Am J Trop Med Hyg* **77**, 289–295 (2007).

276. Aponte, J. J. *et al.* Safety of the RTS, S/AS02D candidate malaria vaccine in infants living in a highly endemic area of Mozambique: a double blind randomised controlled phase I/IIb trial. *Lancet* **370**, 1543–1551 (2007).

277. Olotu, A. *et al.* Four-year efficacy of RTS, S/AS01E and its interaction with malaria exposure. *N Engl J Med* **368**, 1111–1120 (2013).

278. Wipasa, J. and Riley, E. M. The immunological challenges of malaria vaccine development. *Exper Opin Biol Ther* **7**, 1841–1852 (2007).

279. Epstein, J. E. *et al.* Safety and clinical outcome of experimental challenge of human volunteers with Plasmodium falciparum-infected mosquitoes: an update. *J Infect Dis* **196**, 145–154 (2007).

280. Hoffman, S. L. *et al.* Protection of humans against malaria by immunization with radiation-attenuated Plasmodium falciparum sporozoites. *J Infect Dis* **185**, 1155–1164 (2002).

281. Luke, T. C. and Hoffman, S. L. Rationale and plans for developing a non-replicating, metabolically active, radiation-attenuated Plasmodium falciparum sporozoite vaccine. *J Exp Biol* **206**, 3803–3808 (2003).

282. Daubenberger, C. A. First clinical trial of purified, irradiated malaria sporozoites in humans. *Expert Rev Vaccines* **11**, 31–33 (2012).

283. Seder, R. A. *et al.* Protection against malaria by intravenous immunization with a nonreplicating sporozoite vaccine. *Science* **341**, 1359–1365 (2013).

284. Good, M. F. Immunology. Pasteur approach to a malaria vaccine may take the lead. *Science* **341**, 1352–1353 (2013).

285. Kaiser, J. Infectious diseases. Unconventional vaccine shows promise against malaria. *Science* **341**, 605 (2013).

286. Matuschewski, K., Hafalla, J. C., Borrmann, S. and Friesen, J. Arrested Plasmodium liver stages as experimental anti-malaria vaccines. *Hum Vaccin* **7**, Suppl: 16–21 (2010).

287. Vaughan, A. M., Wang, R. and Kappe, S. H. Genetically engineered, attenuated whole-cell vaccine approaches for malaria. *Hum Vaccin* **6**, 107–113 (2010).

288. Aly, A. S., Lindner, S. E., MacKellar, D. C., Peng, X. and Kappe, S. H. SAP1 is a critical post-transcriptional regulator of infectivity in malaria parasite sporozoite stages. *Mol Microbiol* **79**, 929–939 (2011).

289. Spring, M. *et al.* First-in-human evaluation of genetically attenuated Plasmodium falciparum sporozoites administered by bite of Anopheles mosquitoes to adult volunteers. *Vaccine* **31**, 4975–4983 (2013).

290. Good, M. F. *et al.* Cross-species malaria immunity induced by chemically attenuated parasites. *J Clin Invest* (2013). doi: 10.1172/JCI66634

291. Pombo, D. J. *et al.* Immunity to malaria after administration of ultra-low doses of red cells infected with Plasmodium falciparum. *Lancet* **360**, 610–617 (2002).

292. Stanisic, D. I., Barry, A. E. and Good, M. F. Escaping the immune system: how the malaria parasite makes vaccine development a challenge. *Trends Parasitol* **29**, 612–622 (2013).

293. Sedegah, M., Hedstrom, R., Hobart, P. and Hoffman, S. L. Protection against malaria by immunization with plasmid DNA encoding circumsporozoite protein. *Proc Natl Acad Sci USA* **91**, 9866–9870 (1994).

294. Doolan, D. L. and Hoffman, S. L. The complexity of protective immunity against liver-stage malaria. *J Immunol* **165**, 1453–1462 (2000).

295. Doolan, D. and Hoffman, S. L. Nucleic acid vaccines against malaria. *Chem Immunol* **80**, 308–321 (2002).

296. Wang, R. *et al.* Boosting of DNA vaccine-elicited gamma interferon responses in humans by exposure to malaria parasites. *Infect Immun* **73**, 2863–2872 (2005).

297. Rogers, W. O. *et al.* Protection of rhesus macaques against lethal Plasmodium knowlesi malaria by a heterologous DNA priming and poxvirus boosting immunization regimen. *Infect Immun* **70**, 4329–4335 (2002).

298. Weiss, W. R. *et al.* Protection of rhesus monkeys by a DNA prime/poxvirus boost malaria vaccine depends on optimal DNA priming and inclusion of blood stage antigens. *PLoS ONE* **2**, e1063 (2007).

299. Li, S. *et al.* Viral vectors for malaria vaccine development. *Vaccine* **25**, 2567–2574 (2007).

300. Chuang, I. *et al.* DNA prime/Adenovirus boost malaria vaccine encoding P. falciparum CSP and AMA1 induces sterile protection associated with cell-mediated immunity. *PLoS One* **8**, e55571 (2013).

301. Sedegah, M. *et al.* Sterile immunity to malaria after DNA prime/adenovirus boost immunization is associated with effector memory CD8+T cells targeting AMA1 class I epitopes. *PLoS One* **9**, e106241 (2014).

302. Ewer, K. J. *et al.* Protective CD8+ T-cell immunity to human malaria induced by chimpanzee adenovirus-MVA immunisation. *Nat Commun* **4**, 2836 (2013).

303. Hodgson, S. H. *et al.* Evaluation of the efficacy of ChAd63-MVA vectored vaccines expressing circumsporozoite protein and ME-TRAP against controlled human malaria infection in malaria-naive individuals. *J Infect Dis* **211**, 1076–1086 (2015).

304. Limbach, K. J. and Richie, T. L. Viral vectors in malaria vaccine development. *Parasite Immunol* **31**, 501–519 (2009).

Index

A

acetyl pyridine NAD, 48
acidic terminal sequence (ATS), 159
acquired immunity, 67
acridine orange, 168
actin–myosin motor, 117
Adams, John, 121
adenovirus (Ad), 227
adenovirus/pox virus platform, 142
adjuvant, 68–70, 74, 86
Aedes, 9, 14
aestivo-autumnal malaria, 5
Affymax Research Institute, 158
Agouron Institute, 90, 97
Albach, Richard, 35
Alfalfa mosaic virus (AMV), 187
Alger, Nelda, 81
Allee, W. C., 26
Allred, David, 165, 171
American Institute of Biological
   Sciences (AIBS), 87–88
Anders, Robin, 137–138
Anderson, John, 30
anemia, 22–23
anion transporter, 166

Anopheles gambiae genome, 113
Anopheles, 9, 16–17, 173–175
antibody-dependent cellular
   inhibition (ADCI), 147, 149
anti-gamete immunity, 179–181
antigenic variation, 153–156, 158, 165
Aotus monkey, 64, 84–89, 96–97,
   134, 167, 169
apical membrane antigen 1 (AMA-1),
   135, 139–141, 226–228
ASO2A (an oil in water emulsion
   containing 3-deacylated
   monophosphoryl lipid A and QS21,
   a saponin-like adjuvant), 134
AT-rich genome, 111

B

B lymphocyte, 125–126
Babesia bovis, 139
Bacillus malariae, 1
bacteriophage vector, 137
bacteriophage, 101–102
Ball, Gordon, 52
Ballou, Ripley, 210, 213
Bancroft, William, 108

band 3 protein, 166–170
Barnwell, John W., 156–157
Barr, Mary, 81
Barrell, Bart, 106
Bastianelli, Giuseppe, 15, 17, 152
Beale, Geoffrey, 176
Becker, Elmer, 204
Behring, Emil von, 71
Belser, William (Bill), 51
Benenson, Abram S., 204
benign tertian malaria, 23
Berghe, Louis van den, 192
Berriman, Matt, 113–114
Bignami, Amico, 5, 13, 15, 17, 152
Bill & Melinda Gates Foundation,
    163, 213, 217
Biomedical Research Institute, 90
bird malaria, 6, 11, 14, 17–18, 31, 33,
    44, 73
Blackman, M. J. (Mike), 130
blood stage vaccine, 67, 89, 115,
    134
blood-stage antigen, 81, 91, 132
Bordet, Jules, 71
Borneo fireback pheasant, 55
Bovell, Carlton, 51
Brown Jr, Frank A., 32, 35
Brown, Harold, 119
Brown, Ivor, 154
Brown, Neil, 60, 153–156, 166
BS3 (bis-(sulfosuccinimidyl)
    suberate), 168–169
Buck, John, 30
Bueding, Ernest, 45
Bullock, Theodore, 30
Burns, Jim, 131
Burroughs Wellcome Fund, 108, 110,
    113
Butcher, Geoffrey, 79, 119

C
Camus, Daniel, 123, 207
candle jar, 65
Caporossi, Theresa, 43
Carlton, Jane, 112
Carter, Henry Van Dyke, 5
Carter, Richard, 176–177, 180–181,
    184
Carucci, Daniel, 107–108
complementary DNA (cDNA), 103
Celera Genomics, 104–105, 111–112,
    216
cell-free protein synthesizing system,
    61
Celli, Angelo, 3–4
Center for Clinical Vaccinology, 227
cerebral malaria (CM), 24, 160
Chaikelis, Alexander, 29
Chemotherapy of Malaria
    (CHEMAL), 61, 164–165
Chen, David, 179, 181
chimpanzee Adenovirus 63
    (ChAd63), 227–228
Chitnis, Chetan, 121
chondroitin sulfate A (CSA), 162–164
chondroitin sulfate, 160
Christophers, Rickard, 174
chromosome, 110–112
chromosome-by-chromosome
    shotgun sequencing, 110
Ciba Foundation, 138
CIDRα1, 161
circumsporozoite protein (CSP),
    193–194, 199, 201, 207, 211, 217,
    220, 226–229, 232
City College of New York (CCNY),
    25–30, 191
Clark, Ian, 128
Cleveland L. R., 42

Clostridium tetanae, 71
Cluster of differentiation 36 (CD36),
    159–161, 163, 168
Clyde and Rieckmann, 216
Clyde, David, 195–198
Coggeshall, Lowell T., 55, 70
Cohen, Joe, 79, 82, 146, 211–212
Cohen, Sydney, 78, 83, 119, 135, 155
Collins, Bill, 167
Collins, Francis, 105
Colombian Malaria Institute, 88
complementary base pairing,
    100–101
complementary DNA (cDNA)
    expression library, 102
Computational Biology Branch
    (CBB), 112
continuous culture, 65–66
Cota-Robles, Eugene, 50
Councilman, W. T., 5
Cowman, Alan, 105, 139–140, 221
Cox, R. A. (Bob), 60, 61
Craig, Alistair, 105
Crick, Francis, 99
Crandall, Ian, 166–167, 171
Cross, George A. M., 128–130
CS gene, 200, 208, 210
Culex, 9, 14, 17
culture system, 206
Cummings, Leda, 111–112
cysteine-rich interdomain region
    (CIDR), 159
cytoadherence, 153, 169

D

D'Alesandro, Philip, 43, 48–49
D'Antonio, Lawrence, 81
Daly, Tom, 132
Dame, John, 112, 208

Davis, Ronald, 137
Dawson, James, 26
DBL2, 164
DBL4, 164
DBL5, 164
DBR synthetic peptide, 170
DIDS binding region (DBR), 164,
    167–169
de Kruif, Paul, 38, 40–41
Deans, Judith, 135–136
dense granules, 75, 117
Department of Biology, 35–36
Department of Defense, 113
Desowitz, Robert, 119, 162
Diaz, George, 88
dichloro-diphenyl-trichloroethane
    (DDT), 174, 177
DIDS (4, 4′ diisothiocyano-2,
    2′-stilbenesulfonic acid), 167
Diggs, Carter, 91, 203–207, 209
Dionisi, Antonio, 15
DNA duplication, 100
DNA plasmids, 225
DNA polymerase, 100, 103
DNA sequencing, 105
DNA-based vaccines, 225
DNAX, 158
Druilhe, Pierre, 147
Duffy antigen, 123
Duffy Binding Proteins (DBPs), 115
Duffy binding-like (DBL), 159
Duffy factor antigen, 120
Duffy negative, 120–121
Duffy positive, 120
Duffy, Patrick, 162–163

E

Eaton, Monroe D., 70, 154
Eda, Shigetoshi, 171

EE form, 21
Ehrlich, Paul, 72
Ellis, Joan, 200
En (a−) cells, 122
Enders, John, 93–94
endothelial protein C receptor
    (EPCR), 160
endothelial receptors, 168
Engerix-B, 213
enzyme heterogeneity, 45
Erickson, James M., 87–88, 91
EBA-175 (erythrocyte binding
    antigen 175), 122–125, 148, 207
erythrocyte binding proteins (EBPs),
    121
erythrocytic schizogony, 22
Espinal, Carlos, 87–88
Etkin, William, 29
exflagellation, 5
exoantigens, 148, 206
EE (exo-erythrocytic), 18–20, 220
expressed sequence tags (ESTs),
    104
Eyles, Don E., 177

F

Fairley, Neil, 19
Falciparum Culture Rockefeller
    (FCR-3), 65, 96
Falciparum Vietnam Oak-Knoll
    (FVO), 13, 15–18, 64, 159, 173
Falciparum Uganda Palo Alto (FUP),
    84–85
Farley, Patrick, 132
Flexner, Simon, 39
flow vial, 65
FMP1/AS02A, 91, 130
FMP2.1/ASO2A, 141

Franklin, Rosalind, 99
Freeman, Robert (Robbie), 128–130
French, Sarah L., 106
Freund, Jules, 67–69, 73–74
Freund's complete adjuvant (FCA),
    74, 82–83, 85–86, 234
Freund's incomplete adjuvant (FIA),
    82, 96
Fried, Michal, 162–163
Friedl, Frank, 30, 37
Friedman, Milton, 65
FSV-1, 208, 210, 217

G

Gambian serum, 78–79
GAO investigation, 90
GAO report, 91
Gardner, Malcolm, 107–108, 111–113
Garnham, P. C. C. (Cyril) , 20, 179
Geiman, Quentin M., 84–85
gene expression libraries, 102
Genentech, 201
General Accounting Office (GAO),
    88, 209
Genetically Attenuated Parasites
    (GAPs), 219–222
genetically attenuated sporozoites, 223
Gengou, Octave, 71
genomic DNA library, 102
Gerhardt, C., 3
Gerrick International, 88
GlaxoSmithKline (GSK), 91, 201,
    208, 210–211, 213–214
Global Malaria Eradication Program,
    79
glutamate-rich protein (GLURP), 148
glycophorin A, 123
GMZ2, 148–149

Godson, Nigel, 200
Golgi, Camillo, 4
Good, Michael, 223
Goodwin, Patricia, 110
Grassi, Giovanni Battista, 13–18, 173
Groman, Neal, 51
Gruenberg, Jean, 165, 171
guanine plus cytosine (G+C), 56
Gumpf, David, 166
Guthrie, Neil, 167, 171
Gwadz, Robert, 177–178, 180, 200
Gysin, Jurg, 167

H

Hand, Cadet, 30
Hadley, Terence, 123, 207
Haemoproteus, 6
Hall, Neil, 113–114
Hawking, Frank, 154
Haynes, David, 206
Heidelberger, Michael, 72–73, 205, 222
hemozoin, 2–4, 22, 36–37
Heppner, Gray, 211–213
herd immunity, 175
Herrera, Socrates, 144, 170
Higginson, Betty, 61
Hockmeyer, Wayne, 208
Hoffman, Stephen L., 106–108, 112, 210, 215–219, 225
Holder, Anthony P., 105, 129–132
Hollingdale, Michael, 90
Honigberg, Bronislaw, 35
Hotchkiss, Rollin, 55
Howard, James, 128
Howard, Randall, 97
Howard, Russell J., 157–159, 165–166

HPLQKTY (= histidine–proline–leucine–glutamine–lysine–threonine–tyrosine), 167–170
HRP (see histidine-rich protein), 75
Huff, Clay, 19, 31–32, 34–36, 38
Hull, Robert, 30–32, 34–36, 38
Human Genome Project, 104–105
hybridoma, 126–127
Hyman, Libbie, 26
hypnozoites, 20, 23
hypothetical proteins, 114

I

ICAM-1, 160
Ilan, Joseph, 59, 61
immune serum, 70–72, 79, 97
in vitro cultures, 95
Institute for One World Health, 217
irradiated cercaria, 191
irradiated sporozoite, 190, 195
isoenzymes, 46, 176

J

Jackson, George, 48
Jacobs, Henry R., 67
James, Sydney Price, 19–20, 174
Jenner, Edward, 71
Jensen, James B., 64–65, 95
Jones, Lynn, 61

K

Kaplan, Nathan, 47–48, 180
Kappe, Stefan, 219, 221
Karush, Fred, 131
Kaslow, David C., 162, 185–186
Kelsch, Achille, L. F., 2
Kemp, David, 105, 136–137, 139

Kennedy J. R., 170
Kilejian, Araxie, 74–76, 95
Killick-Kendrick, Robert, 179
King, Robert C., 32–33, 35
Kitasato, Shibasaburo, 71
Klebs, Edwin, 1, 71
Klots, Alexander, 191
Klotz, Irving M., 33
knob, 153, 165–166
knowlesi ribosomes, 61
Koch, Robert, 16–17, 40, 68–69, 71, 77
Kohler, Georges, 126
Krotoski, W. A., 20
Kudo, R, 31
Kunkel, Henry G., 46–47

L

Lackey, James, 27–28
lactate dehydrogenase (LDH), 46, 48
Langreth, Susan, 91, 95, 153
Laveran, Alphonse, 4–6, 8, 14, 68
Leech, James H., 157
Lewis, Sinclair, 40
ligase, 101
Ling, Irene, 131
Lips, Marcel, 191–192
Loeb, Jacques, 40
Loeffler, Friedrich, 71
Lofton, Susan, 89
Long, Carole, 131
Lophurae igniti igniti, 55
Lorand, Lazlo, 33
Lynch, Clara, 33

M

MacCallum, William, 6, 68
Malaria Genome Project, 107, 109
malaria parasite chromosomes, 105

malaria pigment, 8, 23, 45
Malaria Vaccine and Immunology
    Research (MVIR), 87, 91, 208–209
Malaria Vaccine Development
    Program (MVDP), 91, 209
Malaria Vaccine Initiative (MVI), 92,
    186, 213
Malaria Vaccine Rainbow Tables,
    228
malignant malaria, 5
malignant tertian malaria, 23
Malstat, 48
Manson, Patrick, 7–8, 13–14
Marchiafava, Ettore, 3–4
Marine Biological Laboratory (MBL),
    29, 37, 52, 55, 151
Marmur, Julius, 45, 48, 55–56
Maxygen, 159
Mayer, Manfred, 72
McBride, Jana, 130
McCutchan, Tom, 208
McDonald, Vincent, 75, 171
McGhee, Barclay, 117–118
McGregor, Ian, 78–79, 146, 155,
    191
Meckel, Heinrich, 2
Medawar, Peter, 60
Medical Research Council (MRC),
    119
Menard, Robert, 220
merogony, 22
merozoite antigen(s), 79, 96, 130
merozoite invasion, 117–119, 122,
    142–143, 234
merozoite surface antigen, 97
merozoite surface protein 3 (MSP-3),
    91, 139, 142, 145, 147–148, 228, 232
merozoite surface protein-119
    (MSP-119), 131–132, 134

merozoite surface protein-142,
(MSP-142), 134–135, 226
merozoites, 22–23, 81–83, 85, 96,
116–117
Merrifield, Bruce, 144
Meyers, Gene, 105
microgamete immobilization reaction,
179
microgametes, 22
micronemes, 116, 121
Miller, Jr, Oscar L., 106
Miller, Louis H., 118–119, 121, 123,
157–158, 176–178, 207
Milstein, Cesar, 125
Mitchell, Graham F., 83, 96, 119,
136, 157
Monoclonal Antibodies and Merozoite
Surface Protein (MSP)-1, 125, 128,
130, 132, 134–135
monoclonal antibody, 126–129,
131–132, 136, 166, 182, 184, 207
Moskowitz, Roslyn, 29
Most, Harry, 192, 194, 200
Moulder, James, 34
mRNA, 102
Mudd, Brian, 54
Mulligan, H. W., 189, 193
multiple epitope-thrombospondin
related antigenic protein
(ME-TRAP), 228
Multistage DNA Vaccine Operation
(MuStDO), 225
muramyl dipeptide (MDP), 86, 96
myelomas, 126

N

N-acetylneuraminic acid, 122
NANP, 201–202, 211

National Center for Biotechnology
Information (NCBI), 112
National Institute for Medical
Research (NIMR), 60–61, 107,
130
Naval Medical Research Center
(NMRC), 106, 110–112
Naval Medical Research Institute
(NMRI), 84, 92, 106, 215, 225–227
New York University (NYU),
199–201, 216
Newbold, Chris, 105, 156–158, 165
Newell, Irwin M., 49–50, 52
nicotinamide adenine dinucleotide
(NAD), 48
Night owl monkeys, 84
Nocolaier, Arthur, 71
Northwestern University, 30, 33–36,
38, 52
Novy, Frederick G., 40
Nussenzweig, Ruth, 95, 192,
194–195, 199, 207
Nussenzweig, Victor, 200–201, 220
Nwuba, Roseangela, 130
NYVAC-Pf7, 185

O

Office of Inspector General (OIG), 89
Ogilvie, Bridget, 105
Ogun, Sola, 131
oocysts, 12, 22
ookinete antigens, 185
ookinete surface proteins, 184
ookinete, 6, 22
Opie, Eugene, 6, 46, 68
OptiMal, 48
Oscillaria malariae, 3–4
Osler, William, 5

owl monkeys, 87–88

P

P. berghei, 193, 199, 220
P. chabaudi, 112, 223–224
P. circumflexum, 32
P. cynomolgi sporozoites, 194
P. cynomolgi, 20, 178, 195
P. falciparum (FVO, 3D7 and HB3), 141
P. falciparum cDNA, 138
P. falciparum chromosomes, 106
P. falciparum Erythrocyte Membrane Protein 1 (PfEMP1), 156, 158, 160–161, 165, 168, 171
P. falciparum Genome Project, 111, 114
P. falciparum reticulocyte binding-like homolog protein (PfRH5), 121, 142
P. falciparum sporozoite, 196
P. falciparum, 5, 19–20, 23, 56, 64–66, 79, 81, 84–85, 106–107, 130, 139, 142, 157–158, 160, 167, 221
P. gallinaceum, 32, 145, 177–180, 184, 189–190
P. knowlesi merozoites, 119–120
P. knowlesi sporozoites, 195
P. knowlesi, 22, 61, 70–71, 73–74, 79, 82–84, 116, 121, 136, 154, 156–157, 184
P. kochi, 20
P. lophurae DNA, 56
P. lophurae, 32, 42, 44–46, 48, 53, 55, 63, 67, 69, 74–75, 117, 146
P. malariae, 4, 22–23, 78
P. ovale, 20
P. relictum, 14
P. vivax, 4, 18–20, 23, 72, 120–123, 184
P. yoelii, 112, 128–131, 220–221
P36, 220
P52, 220
Park, Orlando, 35
passive immunity, 72
Pasteur, Louis, 1
Patarroyo, Manuel Elkin, 143–145
pBR322, 137
Pf52/Pf36, 221
Pfalhesin, 164, 167–168
PfGAP vaccine, 222
PfGAP, 221
Pfs230, 182–183
Pfs25, 185–187
Pfs28/Pfs25, 183
Pfs48/45, 182–183, 185
PfSPZ, 215, 217–219
Pg26, 184–185
Pgs25, 182
Pgs28, 183
Pk66, 136
PkDBP, 121
plasmid, 101–102, 227
Plasmodium erythrocyte membrane protein 1 (PfEMP1), 139
Plasmodium genome, 113
Plimmer H. G., 8
PMMSA, 130
polymerase chain reaction (PCR), 102
Potter, Michael, 127
precipitins, 57
Pregnancy malaria (PM), 161–164
premunition, 145–147
prime-boost, 233
Program for Appropriate Technology in Health (PATH), 186, 213
Ps230, 184
Ps25, 185

Ps28, 185
Ps48/45, 184
PvDBP (PvRII), 122
PvDBP, 121
Pvs25, 186

Q

QS21 (a proprietary GSK saponin derivative from the Chilean soap bark tree), 212
quartan malaria, 23
Quillaja saponaria (AS02), 212

R

radiation-attenuated sporozoites, 216
Ravetch, Jeffrey, 105
Read, Clark, 30
recombinant DNA techniques, 101–102, 138
recrudescence, 20
red blood cell membrane receptor, 119
Reese, Robert, 90, 95–97
relapse, 20
RESA, 140
Research Institute of Molecular and Cellular Biology, 158
restriction enzymes, 101–102
RH5-interacting protein, 142
rhoptry, 116
ribosomal protein, 75
ribosome, 59–61, 101
Rieckmann, Karl, 83, 196, 198
Riley, Eleanor, 130
RLF vaccine, 211
RNA polymerase, 101
Robbins, Frederick, 93
Rockefeller Foundation, 174

Rockefeller Institute, 33, 38–39, 41, 43, 45–46, 48, 63, 93–94, 117
Rockefeller University, 74, 95, 130, 144
rocker flask, 64
Rockstein, Morris, 30
Roman Campagna, 16, 19
Ross, Ronald, 6–15, 17–18, 173
Rous, Peyton, 46
Roux, Emile, 40, 71
Rozeboom, Lloyd, 192
RPMI 1640 medium, 64–65
RTS, S, 201–202, 209, 212–214
RTS, S/AS02, 212
Rubin, Gerald, 140
Russell, Paul F., 189–190, 193

S

Sadun, Elvio, 58, 119, 203, 205–206
Saimiri, 87–88, 167, 169
Saint, Robert, 137
Sanaria, 216–217, 219
Sanger Centre, 105, 109–111
Sanger, Frederick, 103
S-antigen, 140
Schaudinn, Fritz, 18–19
Schenkel, R., 81
schizont-infected cell agglutination (SICA), 153–154, 156–157
Schneiderman, Howard, 30
Scripps Research Institute, 97
Seder, Robert, 218–219
senescent red blood cells, 169
sequestration, 64, 152–153, 158–162, 165, 169
Sergent, Edmund and Etienne, 145
Shakespeare, Peter, 60
Shortt, Henry E., 20, 119
sialic acid, 122

Siddiqui, Wasim A., 64, 84–87, 89–90
Silverman, Paul, 64, 79–83, 215
Sinden, Robert, 179
Simpson G., 81
Smith, Edgar A., 81, 87
Sokoyi, Mary, 43
SPf66, 143–144
Spieth, Herman T., 26, 49–50
sporozoite antigen, 198–199
sporozoite asparagine-rich protein 1
    (SAP1), 221
sporozoite vaccination, 190
sporozoites, 19, 21–22, 192
squirrel monkeys, 88
S–s– U (–) red cells, 122
Stanley, Harold, 95, 97
starch block electrophoresis, 46
starch gel electrophoresis, 46
Stauber, Leslie, 57
stearoyl-MDP, 86
Stephens, Grover, 30
Sternberg, George, 1, 4
Stoll, Norman R., 37
sulfadoxine–pyrimethamine, 161
Sulston, John, 109
Sussman, Maurice, 35

T

Takahashi, Yuzo, 152, 171
Taliaferro, William Hay, 32, 57
Tavolga, William, 26
t-butyl hydroperoxide, 169
telomeres, 158
tertian malarias, 23
Tettelin, Herve, 111–112
Thamnomys, 192
The Institute for Genomic Research
    (TIGR), 104, 106–112, 114
therapy by malaria, 19

Thomas, Alan, 135–136
thrombospondin (TSP), 160, 168
thrombospondin related antigenic
    protein (TRAP), 220, 226,
    228–229
Tiffany, Lewis H., 35
Ting, Irwin, 54
Tommasi-Crudeli, Corrado, 1
Tn red blood cells, 122–123
toxin-neutralizing substance, 71
Trager, William, 37–39, 42–47, 49,
    55–56, 63, 65, 85, 93–95, 118,
    144–145
Trager–Jensen cultures, 96, 206, 222
Training in Tropical Diseases (TDR),
    164
transmission control, 173–176
transmission-blocking antibodies, 183
transmission-blocking immunity,
    180–182, 184–185
transmission-blocking vaccine (TBV),
    175–176, 181, 183–185, 187
Trigg, Peter, 60–61
Truong, Father Hoang Quoc, 31
tuberculin, 68–69

U

ultraviolet-irradiated sporozoites,
    189
United Nations Relief and
    Rehabilitation Administration
    (UNRRA), 174
United States Agency for
    International Development
    (USAID), 64, 81–92, 95, 98, 175,
    201, 208–209
University of California at Riverside
    (UCR), 49
University of Florida, 26–28, 30

University of Hawaii, 85, 89–90
University of Oxford, 227
up-regulated in infectious sporozoites
 (UIS), 220
USAID Malaria and Immunology and
 Vaccine Research Program, 98
USAID Malaria Immunology and
 Vaccine Research (MIVR), 81

V

Vac-4-All, 146
Vaccine Research Center (VCR),
 218
Vaidya, Akhil, 131
Vanderberg, Jerome, 191–195, 197
var (variant) genes, 158
var2csa gene, 163
var2csa, 164
Venter, Craig, 104, 106–109, 111–112
Vesell, Elliot, 46–47
Vincke, Ignace, 191–192
virus vectors, 226
Voge, Marietta, 52

W

Walliker, David, 112
Walsh, Charles, 56
Walter and Eliza Hall Institute
 (WEHI), 105, 136–138, 157, 165,
 221
Walter Reed Army Institute of
 Research (WRAIR), 58–59, 91, 119,
 123, 190, 202–208, 210–212, 215
Warren, Leonard, 151
Watson, James, 99
Watterson, Ray, 32, 35–36
Weidanz, William, 131

Wellcome Foundation, 128
Wellcome Trust Genome Campus, 105
 108–109, 113
Wellde, Bruce, 206
Weller, Thomas, 93–95
Wilkins, Maurice, 99
Williamson, James (Jim) , 60
Wilson, Alan, 47–48
Wilson, Iain, 60
Winograd, Enrique, 166
World Health Assembly (WHA), 175
World Health Organization (WHO),
 77, 79, 95, 119, 164, 174
Wright, Kenneth, 50

X

x-irradiated mosquitoes, 192,
 194–196
x-irradiated sporozoites, 193–194,
 198–199, 206, 215, 217, 233–234

Y

Yersin, Alexandre, 71
YETFSKLIKIFQDH (= tyrosine–
 glutamic acid–threonine–
 phenylalanine–serine–lysine–
 leucine–isoleucine–lysine–
 isoleucine–phenylalanine–
 glutamine–aspartic acid–histidine),
 167–170
Yoeli, Meier, 192

Z

zanzarone, 16
Zinsser, Hans, 94
Zolg, Werner, 90
Zuckerman, Avivah, 57–58